3/94

LIB/LEND/001

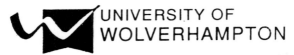

UNIVERSITY OF WOLVERHAMPTON

Dudley Campus Li

Castle View
Dudley DY1

'Volverhampto

D0588802

Antiboo ... ... .tic
AIDS an. society

led at any t
the date
es dis

Tamsin Wilton
with cartoons by the author

UNIVERSITY OF WOLVERHAMPTON
LIBRARY

Acc No.	CLASS
845192	362
CONTROL	11042
DATE SITE	WIL
−4. JUL 1994 D	

WP 0845192 3

WITHDRAWN

New Cl...

for Tom

Contents

Preface

When New Clarion Press asked me whether I would be interested in writing a book about AIDS, my initial reaction was to look at my own bookshelves and the bookshelves in my office at work, both groaning beneath the weight of books about HIV/AIDS, and to say, 'No'. Then I thought about the many people I had met in the course of three years' work in HIV/AIDS training who had asked me to recommend a book which would give them an overview of the different medical and social aspects of the epidemic in plain language, and remembered that even as the specialist literature on AIDS threatens to consume entire forests'-worth of paper, there is actually very little available for the non-specialist. Writing about HIV/AIDS is now a major industry, for the epidemic and its social and political consequences leave few academic disciplines untouched. Medicine, economics, health promotion, gender studies, sexuality studies, cultural studies, political science, sociology, social policy, social work, epidemiology and pharmacology all have their libraries of learned writings about HIV/AIDS. But for the concerned individual who wants to understand not only the scientific facts about the virus, the syndrome and the epidemic but also their social and political significance, there is surprisingly little available. So the first aim of this book is to provide an accessible introduction to the subject for the non-specialist reader. Basic medical information, an overview of some of the major social issues and a potted history of the epidemic are all included, along with a simple guide to safer sex and drug use, information on agencies able to offer advice, information or support, and recommendations for further reading in particular areas of interest.

Sarah Schulman, speaking at the 1990 Outwrite conference in San Francisco, remarked that change happens so rapidly in the field of HIV/AIDS that anyone who writes about the epidemic does so in the knowledge that by the time their words are in print, they will be out of date. This is certainly true of epidemiological statistics and of the specifics of medical research. I have, therefore, not relied heavily on statistics, and this book cannot be an 'up-to-the-minute' account of the exact numbers infected or ill in Britain (or anywhere else). However, I have used recent statistics where to do so enables me to paint a clearer picture of the shape and movement of the epidemic. Readers who want access to the latest figures are advised to contact their local HIV/AIDS organization or the Health Education Authority (see p. 155). The social factors which have played such a powerful part in the spread of the virus do not 'date' in the same way, and the social side to the epidemic which I concentrate on here continues to hold true. Although I do not subscribe to facile notions such as 'human nature' or 'eternal truths', the social aspects of AIDS exist on a much slower time-scale than the medical.

AIDS is, of course, anything but safely confined to the academy. Already (and we are probably still in the early stages of the epidemic), the sad list of those we have lost ranges from the intellectual giant to the children's entertainer. Historians mourn writer Michel Foucault, cineastes have lost critic Vito Russo and film star Rock Hudson, parents and children are bereaved of Muppets creator Jim Henson, photography is diminished by the loss of Robert Mapplethorpe, popular music by the death of Freddie Mercury. Each of us can recite other household names, entertainers, writers, artists, who are known to have HIV or to have died with AIDS.

For many among us, people living with HIV or AIDS and those who are caring for or who have already lost family members, lovers, partners or close friends, the personal significance of AIDS is inescapable. Yet there is still a frightening degree of denial, to the extent that some tabloid journalists still find it possible to fly in the face of overwhelming global evidence and insist that 'normal' people are not at risk. The second aim of this book is to make a realistic appraisal of what the risks are, to expose the political machinations which are largely responsible for ignorance and denial, and to indicate the personal and political strategies needed to bring the epidemic under control. AIDS has been called the epidemic that was allowed to happen; I have tried to expose the ways in which something as fragile and purposeless as this virus has been hijacked in the interests of a variety of political and ideological ends, rather than in the interests of infection control or humanitarian treatment of those infected. This is therefore a campaigning as well as an informative book.

As I slogged my way through the closing pages over the Christmas holiday, I received a Christmas card from a woman I know, a young mother with AIDS. I had not heard from her for months, and was relieved to recognize her writing on the envelope. For many weeks I had been wanting to telephone her but holding back because I was well aware that she might have died, and I was not at all sure that I was ready to mourn the loss of yet another friend to HIV/AIDS. The message in her card explained that she had spent almost all of the past year in hospital. I hope that she will be able to send me a Christmas card next year. The third aim of this book, and for me the most important, is to try to make the world a less vicious and cruel place for the millions of people living with HIV and with AIDS. AIDS may be new but unfortunately human prejudice, bigotry and viciousness are not. People living with the clinical realities of HIV infection have been left to die in corridors or on the street. They have been reviled and stigmatized. Their houses have been burned to the ground. They have been hounded out of their homes and communities, verbally abused and physically attacked. They have lost their jobs, been refused benefits, been forced to beg in the streets. Women with AIDS have been pressured into terminating much-wanted pregnancies. Police have attended AIDS activist demonstrations equipped with (quite unnecessary) rubber gloves, ambulance crews have turned up in 'space suits' to attend people suspected of having HIV, fire-fighters have refused to give mouth-to-mouth resuscitation to anyone they think might be 'at risk'. We are none of us responsible for this virus. But we *are* responsible for the treatment meted out to those with the virus, and we are also, every one of us, responsible for deciding whether to sit back and believe that someone else will 'take care' of HIV/AIDS for us, or to fight back. The epidemic depends on nothing more complex than our own folly for its continued growth. Fighting it demands that we all wake up, wise up and speak up.

I am aware that I could not expect to write about something as sensitive as this epidemic without getting one or two things wrong or making one or two people upset and angry. In some instances I will be quite glad if what I have to say makes certain people angry. My time will be wasted if I have not succeeded in doing that! But I have not intended to be needlessly offensive or unjust, and I have not indulged in malicious misrepresentation. I take full responsibility for any errors. However, nobody ever wrote a book on their own. This one is no exception, and my thanks are due to many people: to Caroline McKinlay for match-making between author and publisher, to Chris Bessant and Fiona Sewell of New Clarion Press for trusting me through what must have been a nail-biting few months, to Lesley Doyal for her friendship and for practical support at a critical moment, to the Terrence Higgins Trust for responding so patiently to esoteric telephone enquiries at unexpected times, and to Stuart for teaching me that even when you are dying, you cannot stop fighting. Most of all I have to thank Ellen Cronin. I know it is traditional for authors to claim they could never have written a word without the love and help of their partner, but in this case it is absolutely true.

Tamsin Wilton

Note on terminology

Throughout the book, I have used terms and expressions which may be unfamiliar to some readers. I have tried to list those here.

HIV stands for *human immunodeficiency virus*, the virus which is associated with AIDS. A person who has HIV may be referred to in many ways, all of which are used at different times in this book. Such a person may be described as *having HIV infection, being HIV positive or HIV antibody positive (HIV+)* or in some contexts simply as *testing positive or being positive.*

HIV infection can give rise to many symptoms and conditions, of which AIDS represents only part. These I refer to as *HIV disease.*

AIDS stands for *acquired immune deficiency syndrome.* Used medically, it refers to a collection of specific opportunistic infections, so called because they seize the opportunity offered by the damage which HIV causes to the immune system to establish themselves in the body of an infected individual. Sometimes such opportunistic infections may be referred to as *AIDS-related illnesses.*

When referring to the physical illnesses linked to HIV and AIDS, I usually refer to *HIV/AIDS*, and when referring to the epidemic I usually refer to the *HIV/AIDS epidemic*, to indicate that, while what is being transmitted in the epidemic is HIV infection, people usually think of the illness associated with HIV infection as AIDS.

When I use *AIDS* on its own, I am usually referring to the cultural and social structure which has grown up around the virus, the imaginary 'AIDS' which has become a shorthand for so much fear, denial and stigma. Thus the 'AIDS industry' or 'AIDS reporting' refer to the social rather than the medical aspect of the epidemic.

You will not find the word 'homosexual' in this book except

where it is impossible or ungainly to substitute anything else. The word is from medical terminology and carries offensive connotations of sickness and abnormality. Additionally, although it refers to both women and men, it has come informally to mean homosexual *man*, thus leaving much room for potential confusion. I therefore use the terms *lesbian* and *gay man*.

The word *homophobia* is also troublesome, since it has come to mean irrational fear and hatred of lesbians and gay men as well as an irrational fear of closeness to members of one's own sex. I do not believe fear and hatred of lesbians and gay men can simply be described as 'irrational' in a culture which so clearly promotes and rewards such hatred. However, there is no obvious alternative, so I use it here to mean simply fear and hatred of lesbians and gay men.

'Heterosexual' is another clumsy term, coined some years after 'homosexual'. It means people who are sexually and emotionally attracted to members of the opposite sex. Depending on context, I sometimes use *heterosexual* and sometimes *straight*.

Heterosexism is the belief that heterosexuality is in every way superior to homosexuality.

1

No longer someone else's problem: the social and medical impact of AIDS

There are young people growing up today for whom AIDS has been around for as long as they can remember, yet for anyone over twenty, it still feels like a relatively new phenomenon. As recently as the late 1970s AIDS and all its associated verbal paraphernalia, 'HIV', 'body positive', 'safer sex', 'needle exchange' etc., were unknown and unimagined. Now it is hard to remember the time when sex seemed, all too briefly, relatively uncomplicated, with the advent of the pill and effective treatments for sexually transmitted diseases. Of course, the apparent simplicity was illusory; sex always retained an element of 'risk', particularly for women; but for two short decades it was at least possible to consign our worst fears to 'the bad old days'.

Now, a 'new' threat has appeared: HIV/AIDS. HIV infection is a global epidemic, and shows little sign of slowing, having spread, in the ten years since it was first identified, to every country in the world. AIDS is now the leading cause of death for women and men aged 20–40 in many major cities in the Americas, Western Europe and parts of Africa, and the World Health Organization (WHO) had been notified of 334,216 cases of AIDS around the globe by the beginning of March 1991. At the end of September 1991, 4,777 men and 288 women were known to have AIDS in the UK, of whom 3,158 had already died.

It is important to remember two things when faced with such statistics. Firstly, AIDS is notoriously underreported in all countries. The inadequate and overstretched health care services of the

1

developing countries mean that people may find it impossible to obtain access to medical care or to a diagnosis; we simply have no means of knowing how many people become ill and die with AIDS without their condition ever being officially recognized or recorded. Another factor which hinders accurate reporting is the stigma which attaches to a diagnosis of AIDS, leading many doctors to avoid mentioning HIV infection or AIDS on death certificates. It is also becoming clear that doctors, just as vulnerable to media misinformation as the rest of us, may simply overlook potential HIV infection in 'untypical' patients, leading again to the possibility of unrecognized and unrecorded AIDS-related deaths, something which is especially true for women, for reasons which will be discussed below. Secondly, cases of AIDS represent no more than the tip of the iceberg of infection. Given an average ten-year symptom-free 'incubation period' for the virus (and up to twenty years not being unknown), during which time an individual may unwittingly infect sexual partners, it is clear that the number of people infected with HIV is very much larger than the number with a clinical diagnosis of AIDS. Just how much larger is a matter for speculation. More conservative estimates suggest that ten people may be infected with HIV for every one person diagnosed with AIDS, but this is widely recognized as a minimum, with other suggestions ranging from twenty to thirty, or even as high as 100. Whatever the hidden reality, it is certain that illness and death will be measured in millions by the end of the decade. The social costs are incalculable.

The story of AIDS is not simply a medical story, for this epidemic casts its shadow over an extraordinarily wide range of human activity, forcing us to question and examine our assumptions and behaviour around issues as diverse as mothering and drug use, sexual activity and health promotion, religious faith and tourism. Perhaps a more positive approach, and the one which informs this book, is to think of AIDS not as a shadow but rather a spotlight which throws the good and the bad in any society into sharp relief. How we, as a society, respond to the challenge of this epidemic is an acid test of our values and our humanity. It is also, clearly, the most rigorous pragmatic test of our social policy, and a unique problem for medical science. So what is this epidemic, at the same time secretive and ruthlessly public, which provokes fear, denial, outrage, hostility and prejudice around the world?

Virus and syndrome

HIV stands for human immunodeficiency virus, and most scientists agree that infection with HIV is what leads to people developing AIDS. AIDS stands for acquired immune deficiency syndrome, and it is *not* a disease. Confusion abounds concerning the relationship between these two, with casual media references to 'the AIDS virus' compounding the problem, and residual doubt remaining in the scientific community about the causal relationship between virus and syndrome.

Viruses have long presented scientific medicine with particular problems. They are very tiny living organisms, responsible for many kinds of human disease, from the common cold and influenza to conditions like herpes, warts and some kinds of cancer. Antibiotics have no effect on viral infections, and the development of anti-viral drugs has proved difficult. One problem is that many viruses mutate rapidly; this is, for example, why influenza seems such a variable disease, with new 'strains' taking hold from time to time with greater or lesser effect. HIV appears to mutate rapidly; it is not uncommon for mutation to be observed during the course of infection in an individual patient, and this clearly poses major problems for those working on vaccines or anti-viral drugs.

HIV is one of the retroviruses, a type of virus whose existence has only comparatively recently been recognized. Retroviruses are like other viruses in that they invade a specific type of body cell; in the case of HIV this is the T helper lymphocyte, a type of blood cell crucially important to the functioning of the immune system. Where they differ from other viruses is in their ability to co-opt the genetic RNA of the host cell in their own reproduction. Once HIV enters a host cell, it may remain inactive for some time (months or even many years) before triggering off the reproduction of new viruses. Once viral reproduction begins, the process kills off increasing numbers of T cells, and it is this which so drastically weakens the body's immune system, leaving the individual vulnerable to a great number of infections, tumours and other illnesses. Frequent T cell counts are generally an important part of medical treatment for people with HIV infection in the developed world, providing a useful marker of the functioning of the immune system, and enabling medication to be given prophylactically (that is, to prevent specific opportunistic infections rather than simply to treat existing ones).

Damage to the immune system

The body responds to infection with any disease-causing organism by producing antibodies. These are usually able to overwhelm the alien cells, but in the case of HIV, the antibodies produced appear to have little effect. Once infected, an individual is infected for life, and it is unlikely that medical science will be able to develop methods of eradicating HIV from the body in the foreseeable future, since anything which damages the virus will of course also damage the blood cells in which it thrives.

The 'symptoms' of HIV infection vary from one person to the next. Many people may notice nothing at all, although there are certain common warning signs. Some people may experience a brief influenza-like illness shortly after infection with HIV. This is known as 'acute HIV infection', and may or may not alert the individual concerned to the possibility of infection. Other common symptoms may follow weeks, months or years later. These can include severe and drenching night sweats, sudden and unexplained weight loss and persistent diarrhoea. Many men (though few women) develop persistent generalized lymphadenopathy (PGL), a swelling of the lymph glands which persists for some time. Apart from damage to the immune system, HIV is also capable of causing damage to the central nervous system. It is able to cross the blood–brain barrier, and sometimes causes encephalopathy (brain disease), resulting in a variety of distressing symptoms which may include memory loss, mood and behavioural changes and a loss of co-ordination or movement problems. But it is the damage to the immune system which most often results in illness or death.

The opportunistic infections

It is a common misconception that people with AIDS are vulnerable to *all* infections; for example, that if someone with AIDS catches a cold, it will kill them. Indeed, AIDS is often presented as an automatic death sentence, a terminal illness. In fact, neither of these is strictly accurate. The immune system is immensely complex, acting on many levels to protect us from disease and illness, and it is not simply 'switched off' by the action of HIV. Rather, one specialized component of the whole system is affected, leaving the greater part of the immune system functioning as normal. It is as if a gardener suddenly found that the greenfly spray had stopped working; the slug bait, fungicide, weedkiller etc. would still be able to rid the garden of slugs, fungi and weeds, but the lack of greenfly spray would mean that the roses would be vulnerable to aphid attack. In much the same way, an immune system damaged by HIV becomes incapable of protecting the body against a specific group of diseases and conditions. Because this part of the immune system has evolved to respond very effectively, most of the conditions which can affect people with HIV-damaged immune systems are either extremely uncommon or usually relatively harmless in people with fully functioning immune systems.

It is this collection of specific diseases and conditions which make up the medical syndrome known as AIDS, and once someone known to be infected with HIV develops one or more of these conditions, they are diagnosed as having AIDS. The list of these so-called 'opportunistic infections' is a long one – over forty recognized medical complaints. These include protozoal infections which can lead to pneumonia, enteritis (inflammation of the bowel) or encephalitis (inflammation of the brain), bacterial infections which can lead to pneumonia, severe diarrhoea or meningitis, viral infections which can cause blindness, pneumonia, skin problems or encephalitis, and fungal infections which can cause meningitis, severe lung disease or inflammation of the digestive tract. They also include some tumours. It is worth focusing on three of the commonest opportunistic infections, Kaposi's sarcoma (KS) – a cancer, candida albicans (thrush) – a fungus, and pneumocystis carinii pneumonia (PCP) – a protozoal infection, to get a fuller idea of the broad spectrum of illnesses which a diagnosis of AIDS can encompass.

KS is a form of skin cancer which, in people uninfected by HIV (when it is called 'classic KS'), is both uncommon and relatively benign, appearing most usually as harmless purplish lesions on the skin of elderly men. In people with AIDS, however, it occurs frequently, and is capable of much greater virulence, spreading much more rapidly through the body and often forming lesions on internal organs, as well as on the skin. When associated with AIDS, it is called 'epidemic KS'. Lesions on the face may be disfiguring and, as they are well known as a 'marker' of AIDS, may give rise to stigma or isolation in communities where HIV infection is relatively common. Lesions on internal organs may cause great pain, internal bleeding, or difficulty in breathing, swallowing etc., depending on the site of the lesions. KS is extremely rare in women with AIDS, for reasons as yet unknown, and incidence among people with AIDS appears to be decreasing as the epidemic progresses, though there are conflicting explanations for why this should be so.

Candida is a fungal infection, familiar to us as a condition which causes white patches in the mouths of babies and young children, or unpleasant vaginal soreness, itching and discharge in women. It is much more common than KS in people without HIV infection, but usually represents more of a nuisance than anything else. For people with AIDS, it can become far more invasive and resistant to treatment, infecting the mouth and the upper digestive tract and making eating painful and difficult.

PCP is a form of pneumonia where the lungs are colonized by protozoa, eventually if untreated causing death by suffocation. It is usually a rare disease of extreme systemic weakness, seen for example in concentration camp survivors after the Second World War, but is relatively common in people whose immune systems have been damaged by HIV. In fact, it was the sudden and unexpected appearance of PCP in 1981, in previously healthy young adults, which first alerted the Center for Disease Control in the USA to what we now recognize as the appearance of AIDS.

Early history of the epidemic

PCP, now identified as one of the classic markers of AIDS, was almost unknown at that time. These first cases of PCP are often referred to as the 'first cases of AIDS', but it would be more accurate to say that they were the first cases of AIDS to be recognized in the USA (and of course, they were not at that time thought of as AIDS at all). As we now know, HIV can remain in the body for a very long time (up to twenty years) before any damage is recognized, so it is probable that the 'new' PCP patients had been infected a long time before they became ill. In fact, the 'first' epidemic of HIV infection probably began in the 1950s, spreading unrecognized during the 1960s and 1970s, soon reaching countries in North America, Europe, Africa and the Caribbean. It was finally recognized in the early 1980s in the United States, as a new and rapidly spreading sickness which at first appeared to be largely confined to young gay men. So convinced was the medical establishment in those early days that male homosexuality somehow *caused* this new epidemic that it was dubbed GRID, Gay-Related Immune Deficiency, a designation which wilfully ignored the known existence of numbers of infected heterosexuals. Even in the USA, AIDS has never been exclusive to gay men, though the gay community was, and continues to be, hard hit by AIDS-related deaths. The pattern in other contexts was very different, often showing dramatic variations over a few hundred miles. For example, in Edinburgh, unsafe injecting drug use was responsible for alarming rates of transmission, while in London the gay male community showed the greatest number of cases, and in sub-Saharan Africa (as is true globally) the mode of transmission has been overwhelmingly through unprotected heterosexual sex. The current trend is of a general steady increase in the rate of heterosexual transmission.

Recently, the notion of 'risk groups' has been replaced by the more accurate and helpful idea of 'risk behaviours'. It is, after all, not who you are but what you do which determines whether or not you will become infected with HIV. Epidemiological statistics which categorize people according to 'risk groups' mask the realities of transmission and lead to a false sense of security. Thus a gay man who may in fact have become infected through drug use, a drug user who became infected through unprotected heterosexual intercourse and a heterosexual man who became infected in Paris even though he regularly travels to central Africa will all end up in misleading and inaccurate categories. Similarly, a gay man who has many sexual partners but always practises safe sex will be at much lower risk than a heterosexual married woman who does not use condoms with her husband because he has not told her about his extramarital affairs.

Because of the long incubation period of this virus, we have been obliged to deal with what appears to be a sudden outbreak on a global scale, but in fact retrospective diagnoses from stored blood and medical records indicate that people in many countries had been dying of what we would now call AIDS as long ago as the late 1950s. HIV and AIDS have been with us for much longer than was originally thought, and there is hardly a corner of the globe untouched. The scale and implications of the epidemic are terrifying. The World Health Organization figures at the end of 1990 showed around 802,000 reported cases of AIDS worldwide, with a further eight and a half million estimated to have HIV. This must be put into perspective. Measles, for example, kills two million children in the developing world every year – four children every minute. But HIV infection is a new disease. It has only been recognized since 1981, but in that time it has cost the United States alone $8.5 billion in health costs, with an additional $55 billion in terms of lost productivity; and it kills one person in the USA every half an hour. At the moment, car accidents still claim more lives than this, but for how much longer will that be true? We do not yet have any means of knowing how much worse it is going to get, but there are certainly no signs that it is getting any better.

But what about the people behind the statistics? What happens to someone who becomes infected?

Full-blown AIDS: a suitable case for treatment

Media coverage gives the clear impression that infection with HIV follows a straightforward linear course, from 'AIDS carrier' to 'AIDS patient' or 'AIDS victim' to 'full-blown AIDS'. This is misleading on several counts. Firstly, not everyone who is infected with HIV will necessarily go on to develop AIDS, something which is increasingly true as treatments are developed to fight the effects of the virus on the immune system. Secondly, AIDS is a syndrome, not a disease, and it cannot be caught or 'carried'. Apart from the fact that it is HIV, not AIDS, which is 'carried' and which may be passed on from one person to another (see below), the phrase conjures up notions of hidden danger, plague and contagion which are quite inappropriate in the context of HIV/AIDS. Similarly, referring to people with AIDS as 'victims' or 'patients' creates the idea of passivity and helplessness, which is not a true reflection of the lives they have to lead. Someone with a diagnosis of AIDS may of course be gravely ill at times, an in-patient in a hospital with all the paraphernalia of medical care. But this is only part of the picture. Effective treatment is available for many of the conditions associated with AIDS, so someone very ill one day may return to work a few weeks later, in good health and quite capable of leading a full and 'normal' life. People with AIDS are best thought of as just that, people first, and 'with AIDS' second. They are engaged in living with AIDS, devising strategies for coping, for surviving, for getting the most out of their lives, and their AIDS diagnosis may in fact play a relatively small part in that life.

Perhaps the most misleading term of all is 'full-blown AIDS'. It creates the impression of a logical progression to a predictable outcome, from which there can be no turning back. One of the unique characteristics of AIDS, and one of the things which marks it out from other potentially terminal conditions, is that it is quite remarkably unpredictable, and no two individuals with a diagnosis of AIDS will experience the same (or even necessarily a similar) pattern. One person infected with HIV may experience no illness at all for many years, and then suddenly and unexpectedly fall ill and die within a few months. This pattern, once extremely common while medical science struggled to find out just what was going on, is now less and less likely, at least for those with access to good medical care. Another may spend eight or ten years on a see-saw of health and illness, alternating between lying in a hospital bed feeling very ill indeed to being up and mobile and feeling perfectly fit and well. Yet another may experience a gradual, but irreversible, decline in health, with little respite from lengthy periods of illness. One person may become blind, another may experience depression and mood changes, yet another may need to use a wheelchair.

It is this characteristic uncertainty which colours much of our social experience of HIV. In the industrialized world we have been lulled into a largely illusory conviction that medical science has managed to 'organize' the body and its illnesses in a logical, predictable way. The medical model of health and disease encourages a linear way of thinking about health; an identifiable 'event' such as infection with a bacterium or falling downstairs causes damage to the body, the patient experiences symptoms, medical technology deals with the cause and/or offers relief of the symptoms, the patient becomes well again. HIV challenges those certainties on every level.

Someone infected with HIV may not experience any symptoms for many years, may perhaps be run over by a lorry before they are ever aware they are infected, yet they may still pass the virus on to others. An individual who is aware that they are infected with HIV can be given little idea of what to expect. What is certain is that disease progression is closely related to early diagnosis, socio-economic factors and access to appropriate medical treatment; people living in deprivation and poverty are more likely to acquire HIV infection in the first place, and once they are infected, to become ill sooner and more seriously, and to die sooner than relatively affluent people. Although people living with AIDS quite rightly insist that they are *living* with the syndrome, not *dying* of it, the fact is that the average time from an AIDS diagnosis to death in the industrialized West is currently about five years for an adult man (though of course many live for much longer and survival time increases all the time as medical care improves). For women, as the ACT UP New York Women and AIDS group point out in their book *Women, AIDS and Activism*, that survival time is halved.

Relative safety: transmission issues

Studies, such as that carried out by the Health Education Authority in 1988 to evaluate their public information campaign, have shown that most people in the UK now know that HIV is spread by unprotected sex, by the medical use of contaminated blood or blood products or by sharing drug-injecting equipment, and from mother to baby. Patterns of transmission differ from country to country and even between regions within countries (see below), but sexual transmission is overwhelmingly the most common, with hetero-sexual intercourse accounting for over 60 per cent of all infections by the early 1990s, a figure which continues to increase.

To be faced with a virus which can infect people without their knowledge and without changing them in any way, and which additionally may be transmitted during that most anxiety-provoking business of sex, is terrifying. We want to know how to protect ourselves, we demand the information we need to keep ourselves safe, deluging safer sex educators with questions: is oral sex safe? what about bondage? can I make love to my girlfriend during my menstrual period? what about couples who have been mutually faithful for seven or eight years? what if we are both virgins?

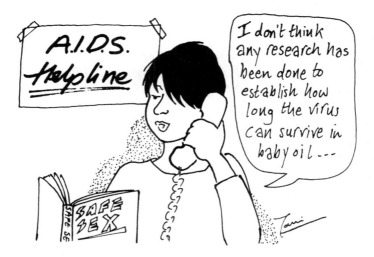

One of the hardest things to accept about this epidemic is that there are very few hard and fast rules about sexual transmission. It is impossible in most cases to say conclusively either that a particular activity is 100 per cent 'safe' or that it will *definitely* result in transmission. A study reported in *AIDS Newsletter* which focused on the wives and girlfriends of haemophiliacs in Australia, who unknowingly continued full sexual lives for some years after their partners were infected with HIV, showed that the transmission rate was unexpectedly low. On the other hand, there are several well-documented cases of young women who have become infected as a result of their first act of intercourse. Cunnilingus appears to be extremely 'safe', but there are a handful of cases where it was the only identified 'risk behaviour' of individuals who became infected. 'Deep' kissing is clearly 'low risk' – there have been no cases of the virus being transmitted in this way; yet the virus *is* found, albeit in small amounts, in saliva, and there is a *theoretical* risk that enough could be transmitted for infection to occur if, for example, one partner had open sores on their lips or gums. To most, that theoretical risk remains in the realm of statistics, assessed quite reasonably as not worth bothering about. To some, who may have a partner known to have HIV, or who may be especially anxious about sex, *any* risk, however slight, is not worth taking.

So what *is* safe sex? We know that the virus is present in infectious quantities in blood, semen and vaginal fluids. We know that, when considering sexual risk, semen appears to be the greatest hazard. Cindy Patton, American author of *Sex and Germs*, one of the first books to address the politics of the epidemic, summarizes her message as 'Don't get semen in your anus or vagina', a simple rule of thumb which has the advantage of applying equally to heterosexuals and gay men. However, it is entirely irrelevant to lesbians, and takes no account of the fact that vaginal fluids may be infectious too, and so women can infect men.

Educators tend to distinguish between *safe* sex, which is sex which does not involve penetration with the penis, and *safer* sex, which involves penetration, but with a condom. 'Safer' simply recognizes that penetration with a condom cannot be called 'safe', because condoms have a habit of breaking, slipping off or leaking. They are, after all, far from 100 per cent effective as contraceptives, and whereas a woman can only get pregnant at certain times during her fertility cycle, there is no such cycle for infection with HIV. In order to make the risk of HIV truly minimal, penetration must be avoided altogether, a far from easy task in a culture which labels anything other than penetration 'not real sex'. Some of the problems with safe and safer sex are discussed in later chapters and in appendix 1.

HIV is best thought of not as a sexually transmitted disease but as a blood-borne virus (like hepatitis B). It is transmissible sexually, since sexual fluids such as semen contain fluids from the blood, but it is also transmitted in other ways which allow blood-to-blood contact. The most important are during pregnancy and childbirth, or during activities which pierce the skin.

Pregnancy and childbirth

It was originally thought that HIV/AIDS had a disastrous effect on childbearing; that HIV infection in a woman would progress more rapidly to AIDS if she became pregnant, that her baby had a high risk of being infected, that breast milk was highly infectious; in short, that women with HIV would be well advised not to have children, and to terminate any existing pregnancy at the time of diagnosis. We now know that there is no convincing evidence that pregnancy exacerbates or hastens illness in women with HIV, that the advantages of breastfeeding far outweigh the small risk of infection to the baby, and that the risk of transmitting HIV to the child in the womb or during birth is probably between 10 and 12 per cent. However, there can be no doubting the painful and complex issues which potentially face a woman who is HIV+ when she is deciding whether or not to become pregnant or to continue a pregnancy, or the unprecedented social costs of infant HIV infection worldwide. In the developing world, the WHO states that, because of the high numbers of babies born with HIV, 'the advances of child-survival programmes of the past 20 years may already be reversed', while in the United States, AIDS is already the ninth leading cause of death among children aged 1 to 4, with 2,500 children diagnosed with AIDS by July 1990 (statistics taken from the Panos Institute's dossier *The Third Epidemic*.

Skin piercing

In the early stages of the epidemic, many people became infected with HIV by receiving blood or blood products containing quantities of the virus. This was how many haemophiliacs in the UK, for example, were infected, as were recipients of blood transfusions.

Blood and blood products are now screened, and the possibility of acquiring HIV infection in this way within the UK is virtually nil. Other procedures, such as vaccination, testing blood, dental injections and treatment, surgery, acupuncture, even tattooing and ear-piercing, all of which represent a *potential* transmission risk for clients and practitioners, are now covered by appropriate guidelines, and infection is extremely unlikely when using reputable practitioners.

Recreational or addictive use of injectable drugs poses a different set of problems. Although it is important to recognize that many injecting drug users have become infected with HIV through sex, it is clear that many have acquired the virus by sharing injecting equipment. Clearly, if two people share injecting equipment and one of them has HIV, it is relatively easy for the virus to contaminate the needle, syringe or other equipment and simply be injected into the bloodstream of the other user. It is therefore extremely important, for the sake of the whole community, that needle exchange facilities should be available to all injecting drug users (see appendix 2).

The 'AIDS test'

Faced with an 'invisible' epidemic, the possibility that anyone may be infected and not know it, there have been many calls for 'AIDS testing', on an individual or a mass basis. What are the issues around testing?

From what has been said already it will be clear that there is no such thing as an 'AIDS test'. A diagnosis of AIDS is only made in very specific medical circumstances, and has nothing to do with any 'test'. What may be tested for is HIV, and even then, the picture is far from straightforward.

Once HIV has entered the bloodstream, the body begins to manufacture antibodies, and these may be detected by a relatively simple test, known as the ELISA (enzyme-linked immunosorbent assay) test. However, there is frequently a significant time lapse between infection and the appearance of antibodies, up to several months in some cases (in fact, it is now known that this period may extend to one or more years in some instances). This period, popularly known as the 'window of uncertainty', means that an individual may test *negative* for antibodies to HIV despite being infected (and infectious). To allow for this, someone who tests negative is asked to return six weeks later for a second test, if they appear to have been at risk, and must abstain from any risky behaviour between tests. Once antibodies have been detected, a follow-up test called the Western Blot test may be done, as confirmation. Taken together, the two tests have a very high degree of accuracy, but the Western Blot is a far more costly and complex procedure (out of the economic reach of many developing nations, for example).

Once someone has tested positive for antibodies to HIV, they may be referred to as 'HIV antibody positive', 'antibody positive' or simply 'HIV positive' (often contracted to HIV+), or may be said to have 'sero-converted'. To challenge the negative stereotypes about HIV and AIDS, people in the USA and UK who have HIV infection have set up a network of self-help and support groups which they named 'Body Positive', reminding outsiders that people who are 'antibody positive' may still feel very positive about their bodies and their lives and may choose to fight their condition with a positive attitude and by taking positive care of themselves. Some people with HIV infection refer to themselves as 'body positive'. People with AIDS generally prefer to be referred to as just that; the contraction to 'PWAs' is increasingly widely used and its use denotes respect for the wishes of those who are living with a diagnosis of AIDS.

When the nature of the window of uncertainty is understood, it becomes obvious that mass HIV testing has no place in controlling the epidemic. Let us consider the example of a mythical state where HIV infection does not exist, and where the government attempts to prevent the epidemic entering the country by forcibly testing everyone entering from abroad. The most accurate medical test imaginable is probably only 90 per cent accurate, so for every hundred people tested, there will be about ten false negatives and false positives. Additionally, other infections, such as malaria, may give a false positive result (this then unrecognized problem was responsible for an initial overestimation of the epidemic in some African countries). The window of uncertainty means that a number of people who may have been recently infected will test negative, despite the fact that the virus may be most infectious in the early stages. Thus, despite the precaution of mandatory testing, dozens of HIV+ individuals will enter the country. Since they have tested negative, they will naturally believe themselves to be at no risk of HIV, and to pose no risk to others, and will see no need to practise safer sex or drug use. Dozens of other people will unnecessarily carry the complexity of worries which a positive test result brings with it. Yet, despite the counterproductivity of testing used in this way, 29 countries currently have laws demanding mandatory testing of one or more categories of visitor or immigrant.

What about the benefits of the test? There are only two useful applications of HIV testing. The first, and most important, is to enable individuals who have contracted HIV infection to receive appropriate medical care and make any necessary changes in their lives. The second is to enable epidemiologists to judge the rate of HIV infection in order to plan health care and social policies appropriately.

There are important negative consequences of taking the test, which need to be weighed carefully against the potential benefits to the individual concerned or to epidemiologists. Anyone who admits to having taken a test for HIV is likely to be refused life insurance and to find it difficult to obtain a mortgage. There is additionally the trauma of a positive test result. A negative result, on the other hand, may also have undesirable consequences in that the individual tested, having had good reason to fear that they may have been infected, may actually become more irresponsible about practising safer sex and/or drug use, either in the temporary euphoria of relief, or through the belief that they must be 'immune' or 'lucky'. Many would argue that, faced with such contradictions, we can best take responsibility during this epidemic by behaving as though we were all potentially HIV+, and that the best time to start looking after your health is right now ... not simply after a positive HIV test.

On the other hand, there are important decisions to be made by anyone who knows they are HIV+, and it is undoubtedly easier to make them before becoming ill. Finding medical practitioners knowledgeable about HIV/AIDS may be crucial in averting illness or prolonging life, and certain welfare benefits may be available to people with a diagnosis of AIDS. (This is especially true in countries without a national health system, such as the USA.) In the early days of the epidemic, when knowing your antibody status did nothing to improve your health, people were advised that there was little point in being tested, and much to lose. Nowadays, at least in the developed nations, medical care has advanced to the extent that prophylactic medication and treatment of opportunistic infections may significantly extend survival time and quality of life. There are, therefore, very good reasons for taking an antibody test if you suspect you may have HIV.

The issue of the anonymous testing of sample populations (women attending antenatal clinics, for example) is fraught with ethical problems. On the one hand it is argued that effective planning of health promotion, health care and welfare services depends on knowing how the virus is spreading through the population. One way of getting this information is to screen blood samples from selected groups for antibodies to the virus. On the other hand, the usefulness of this procedure depends, among other things, on the size of the sample. It is not feasible to provide adequate pre-test and post-test counselling to large groups of people, since these services are very demanding of resources such as time, money and staff, all of which are under considerable stress in the NHS. Clearly it is quite inappropriate to force mandatory testing on people under these circumstances. The only practical way of getting this information, then, is by anonymous screening. This avoids the problem of supporting individuals who test positive, because no-one is told that their blood is being tested in the first place. The problem of obtaining consent in these circumstances is side-stepped by informing people that if their blood is taken for other purposes, it may also be used without their knowledge for anonymous HIV testing. So, if you do not want your blood to be used in this way, you do have the right to refuse when you find yourself in a situation where it might be. However, the ethical questions raised by a procedure which shows how many blood samples in a target group are infected, without offering that information to the individuals concerned and thus enabling them to obtain early medical care and to protect others from infection, are clearly troublesome.

One virus, many issues

Dr Jonathan Mann, founder of the World Health Organization's Global Programme on AIDS, has identified three global AIDS epidemics. The first was the unsuspected, silent spread of HIV from the 1950s to 1981. The second is the highly visible epidemic of AIDS which we are now witnessing. The third is what might be termed the 'social' epidemic, the various reactions of fear, hatred, bigotry, denial and repression with which the peoples of the world have responded. Such reactions dump an unjust burden on people living and dying with AIDS, but they also exert a profound influence on the lives of us all, from the most cherished intimacies of our sexual and familial relationships to the public carousel of party politics. It is the nature of this third epidemic, the 'social' epidemic, which I intend to explore in greater detail here.

2

Fire and brimstone: press coverage of AIDS and its consequences

Unquestionably, anyone who is seriously ill needs looking after. When we are ill we are not only dependent on others for physical care, we are also emotionally vulnerable, as anyone who has experienced the depression that comes with a bad bout of flu can testify. People faced with the possibility of death are even more in need of loving support. Giving this kind of care to the sick is not always easy, whether for overworked and undervalued nurses or for family members or friends, and caring for people who are dying is made doubly difficult in a society such as ours where death is kept so hidden that it is no longer understood as the natural end of us all, but rather a failure of some kind. Illness and death are potent sources of anxiety. When the illness is contagious, threatening to infect the care-givers, anxiety is quite naturally increased, and when the illness is epidemic and deadly, concern for personal safety is likely to overwhelm compassion. Thus, told that a close family member has yellow fever or cholera, the desire to care for the sufferer struggles with the wish to put oneself as far away from the risk of infection as possible.

It is easy to understand and sympathize with such conflicts when the risk is great. The risk of becoming infected with HIV, however, is very small, and is limited to specific contexts; unless you have unprotected sex with someone who is infected, or unless there is direct blood-to-blood contact, infection cannot occur. Even as a result of accidental needlestick injuries (where a needle contaminated with the blood of an infected person jabs a care-giver) the number of incidents where HIV has been contracted by health care workers is surprisingly small. Yet people living with HIV and with AIDS have become social outcasts in a way which is reminiscent of the treatment meted out to people with leprosy or bubonic plague in the Middle Ages. The stigma attached to the condition is so extreme that they and their families and associates have been subject to neglect, ostracism, abuse and even violence. Leigh Rutledge, in his book *Unnatural Quotations*, cites the disturbing case of three young boys who were HIV+ and were admitted to local schools in Arcadia, Florida. An organization calling itself 'Citizens against AIDS in School' mounted a hate campaign which culminated in the boys and their parents being run out of town after their home was gutted by a fire bomb. In the same book we read of a 24-year-old married man with AIDS being kicked and beaten by attackers who claimed they were 'Killing AIDS! And when we've done with you, we're going to kill your wife and kids, just in case they've got it.' The result of such frenzied hatred is to force the added burden of secrecy on to people already faced with the realities of living with HIV/AIDS. Several of the contributors to a British collection of personal accounts entitled *Women Talking About AIDS*, which was published by the charity AVERT, speak about the impossibility of disclosing the nature of their illness to others, their fight to maintain secrecy, and the fear of the isolation, stigma and loss of friends which disclosure would bring.

Additionally, notions of sinfulness and wrongdoing have been associated with HIV/AIDS to a quite remarkable degree. People who discover that they are infected, rather than being offered the support and care they so desperately need, are blamed for their illness. Worse yet, any member of one of the social groups which have been linked with HIV/AIDS in the public mind is liable to find herself or himself accused of *causing* AIDS, and thereby putting 'innocent' people at risk. In addition to coming to terms with an unpredictable and unpleasant medical condition which is likely to kill them, people with HIV/AIDS are faced with anger, hatred, disgust and viciousness where they have a right to expect only care and support. How did this extraordinary and shameful situation arise?

Historically, Western civilizations have responded to mass epidemics by seeking to apportion blame, and by creating scapegoats for that purpose. We seem to be, on a fundamental level, creatures of meaning; we both depend on and endlessly create meaning, often overriding logic in order to do so. It makes us anxious to be faced with something as utterly meaningless as a virus which is capable of wiping out great numbers of (primarily young) people, thereby threatening many of the economic and social structures which we depend upon and around which we organize our lives. It is also, of course, frightening to be faced with the possibility of our own death, and very tempting to seek reassurance that we are in some way able to control that possibility, to avert it. We are eager to believe that 'It won't happen to me.' Since 'it' quite clearly does happen to someone, our security further depends on identifying a likely candidate for extinction, the 'someone else' who represents those at risk while we can reassure ourselves that we do not meet the criteria. We then, of course, have to establish sufficient distinguishing characteristics to enable ourselves (and death) to differentiate between 'us' and 'them', the 'others'. If death stubbornly continues to strike at random, taking individuals from 'our' social group as well as 'them', we may, in order to maintain the fiction which underpins our security, interpret this as direct harm done by 'them', the 'natural victims', to 'us'. The logical corollary of this psychic survival mechanism is that 'they' should be a group which is already hated and feared, and which is seen as disposable in its entirety.

Thus the epidemics of syphilis which raged for centuries were blamed variously on the nationals of any country you happened to be at war with, or on women as a whole (and prostitute women in particular). The first sexually transmitted disease to spread around the world, syphilis, was known as French pox to the English, the Italian disease to the French, Spanish sickness to the Italians and Haitian disease to the Spanish! This xenophobia was not confined to Europe; if you were Russian, you thought of it as Polish sickness, while in Japan it was referred to as Chinese sickness. In cartoon and caricature, syphilis was generally depicted as a woman, usually a prostitute or seductress, and was frequently referred to in popular culture as 'Dame Syphilis'. Blame for the epidemic devastating populations (the disease took a much more virulent form in its early days) was thus mapped on to existing hatreds. Similarly, the early epidemics of bubonic plague, the 'Black Death', were widely blamed on the Jews, who were denounced from pulpit and public house alike as corruption and contagion incarnate. It is chilling, particularly in the context of the homophobia which accompanies AIDS in much of the world, to recall that one of Hitler's justifications for the Holocaust was his identification of syphilis as the 'Jewish sickness'.

Undoubtedly, the 'Jews' in the current epidemic of HIV/AIDS in the USA and Europe are gay men (although it is important to recognize that in other parts of the world, quite different groups, including refugees, tourists, foreign students, prostitutes, 'decadent' Westerners or even scientists, are held to blame). Despite the inescapable fact that it is (unsafe) *heterosexual* intercourse which is (and always has been) the commonest route of HIV transmission globally, and despite steadily increasing rates of HIV infection among heterosexuals in the UK, the link between AIDS and homosexuality seems ineradicable. Much of the responsibility for this damaging state of affairs must be laid at the door of the British press.

The 'gay plague' years

Despite urgent pressure from groups such as the Terrence Higgins Trust (THT) and the Health Education Council (HEC), it was not until 1986, five years after the first AIDS-related deaths in the UK, that the government launched its national public education campaign. Until that time, the only sources of information about HIV and AIDS were press articles, rare television and radio coverage, and the help lines and voluntary groups almost exclusively set up and run by gay men and lesbians. The routine confiscation by HM Customs and Excise of imported gay magazines from the USA meant that the safer sex expertise rapidly developing in the gay community in the States was simply unavailable to anyone in the UK, a factor which has probably resulted in the wanton loss of many lives, both gay and straight.

The British press, not renowned for its liberal or humanitarian

treatment of minorities, set about disseminating 'facts' about HIV/
AIDS which were inaccurate and misleading, and launched into an
all-out attack on homosexuality. 'By 1984', as Zoe Schramm-Evans
commented at the third Social Aspects of AIDS Conference at
London's South Bank Polytechnic, 'the press had all but convinced
a willing public that AIDS was the gay plague.' The perverse and
cruel journalistic legerdemain whereby the group of people in the
developed West *most affected* by the new illness were pilloried as
its *cause* was not limited to the gutter press. On 27 July 1983 an
article in *The Times* declared that 'a network of promiscuous urban
homosexuality, constantly folding back on itself, provides an ideal
diffusion field for any infection getting into it'. The use of pseudo-
scientific terminology such as 'diffusion field' masked blatant
prejudice behind an appearance of detached objectivity; the question as to how 'promiscuous urban homosexuality' might or might
not differ from promiscuous urban heterosexuality (or promiscuous
rural sexualities) was not explored.

The gay-blaming attitude of press reporting of HIV/AIDS takes,
in general, three clearly distinct forms, which may be described as
overt homophobia, covert homophobia, and guilt by differentiation.
The most obvious of these is the grossly offensive overtly expressed
homophobia of the gutter press, which has given rise to some
extraordinarily vicious copy, even by normal tabloid standards.

Overt homophobia

Calls for the isolation or destruction of 'homosexuals' or 'AIDS
suspects' are common, expressed either directly in editorials, or
indirectly though the reported words of others. In this vein, the *Sun*
ran a story (14 October 1985) headlined 'I'd Shoot My Son If He
Had AIDS Says Vicar'. The story was headed up by a dramatic and
disturbing posed photograph of the Reverend Simpson holding a
shotgun to his son's chest, and quoted his sentiments at length.
According to the article, the Reverend 'would ban all practising
homosexuals, who are most in danger of catching AIDS [sic], from
taking normal communion', and he 'calls on the Government to

repeal the law on homosexuality between consenting adults and prostitution, and to punish promiscuity'. He is quoted as saying, 'If it continues it will be like the Black Plague [sic]. It could wipe out Britain. Family will be against family.' The use of the word 'normal' to describe communion is especially telling, implicitly casting 'practising homosexuals' out of the family of the church.

In the same month (3 October 1985), the *Daily Mail* ran an editorial commenting on the American response to AIDS. 'The gay parades are over', it claims. 'So too is public tolerance of a society that paraded its sexual deviation and demanded rights. The public is now demanding to live disease free with the prime carriers in isolation.' Given the enormous and highly public commitment to AIDS prevention and support work which has been shown by the lesbian and gay communities in the USA, this is not only an unapologetic lie, but offensive in the extreme. It also illustrates a strategy almost universal in public statements of this nature in that it excludes lesbians and gay men not only from its assumed readership, but from the 'public' itself. In this piece, 'the public' and 'public tolerance' in fact mean 'heterosexuals' and 'heterosexual tolerance', a piece of linguistic manipulation that would hardly be tolerated were the writer referring to Black or female citizens! Also depressingly familiar is the association of homosexuality with disease, the 'public' apparently hoping to live 'disease free' (an unattainable and unrealistic goal) by isolating 'the main carriers', namely homosexuals (of unspecified gender). The fact that it is heterosexuals who make up the overwhelming majority of those infected in the global epidemic is left unsaid, as is the touchy problem that the isolation of 'carriers' is not only scientifically impossible but would instantly bankrupt any nation attempting the task (Charles Linebarger, writing in 1986 in the USA, is quoted in Simon Watney's book *Policing Desire* as estimating that quarantining everyone testing HIV+ in California alone would cost $7.9 billion, one quarter of the entire annual budget of that state).

Yet this is small beer indeed in comparison to an editorial in the *Daily Star* (2 December 1988) which, beneath the enormous headline 'Ghettos? A Good Idea!', calls for the setting up of 'leper-like colonies', and claims that 'the human race is under threat' from 'promiscuous homosexuals' who 'are by far the biggest spawning ground for AIDS'. It is worth attending to this poisonous piece in some detail, as it has enormous and terrifying implications for the spread of the epidemic. The language is skilfully manipulative; the use of the word 'leper' conjuring up ancient fears of contagion, while phrases such as 'spawning ground' evoke ideas of both unchecked breeding and lower life forms (it is fish, eels and amphibians, all seen as rather slimy and unpleasant creatures, who 'spawn'), thus contributing to an image of homosexuals as base, animal and deeply threatening to 'the human race' by virtue of their 'leper-like' state. Note the ultimate exclusion here; no longer simply content with writing homosexuals out of the 'general public', this piece throws them summarily out of 'the human race' itself! The implications for the prevention of HIV are of course unforgivable. By constructing 'AIDS' (and there is no mention of HIV in this piece) as something associated with promiscuity and homosexuality, both seen as far removed from daily human life, the (putatively heterosexual) reader is led to believe that AIDS is foreign to heterosexuals and that it is, in any case, associated with 'promiscuity'. Rather than encouraging its readership to familiarize themselves with the practice of safer sex and to recognize their own potential risk of HIV infection, the *Daily Star* is inculcating them with the belief that ghettoizing homosexuals is the best way to prevent the epidemic spreading. The word 'homosexual' is used without differentiating between lesbians and gay men, leading to the assumption that it is 'deviant' sex *itself* which is responsible for AIDS. Since lesbians are statistically the group at least risk of HIV infection (cases of woman-to-woman sexual transmission are very rare), it would be infinitely more useful to ask how other groups may learn from lesbian sexual practices in order to reduce their own risk. The very remoteness of the possibility of any such suggestion appearing in the press reveals just how deep-seated are the roots of prejudice in British society.

The virulence of the tabloid attack on gay men reached some sort of ghastly apotheosis on 6 May 1987, when the *Sun*, surpassing its longstanding record as the paper most obsessed with and most hysterical about homosexuality, ran a piece headlined 'Fly Away

Gays – And We Will Pay!', in which it offered free one-way airline tickets to Norway, supposedly to encourage gay men to leave Britain permanently in the public interest. It should not surprise us that, with the openly expressed homophobia of the press setting the agenda in the early years of this epidemic, the unhelpful label 'gay plague' has taken such a hold on the public mind.

Covert homophobia

We have come to expect the tabloids to behave badly, and have a naive faith in the distinction between the 'quality' and the 'gutter' press, comforting ourselves that the 'serious' newspapers are above such dealings, and that we will find minorities represented with tolerance, fairness and even sympathy within their pages. It is indeed true that the standard of reporting is on the whole more balanced, and that the rantings of the tabloids are not to be found in papers such as *The Times*, the *Independent* or the *Guardian*. However, these papers have been known to print directly sensational material, and are the prime offenders when it comes to covert expressions of prejudice against lesbians and gays in their HIV/ AIDS reporting.

Thus, we find in the *Daily Telegraph* (6 November 1985) the headline 'Communion Wine Fears After AIDS Priest Dies', a quite irresponsible slant to the story of a priest's death, labelling the dead man in a way which is clearly stigmatizing and arousing fears about the (non-existent) possibility of contracting HIV/AIDS from the communion chalice. Since it would be just as easy to headline the story 'Communion Wine – Fears Allayed After Priest Dies With AIDS', it is clear that sensationalism has taken editorial priority over responsibility to inform the readership.

In an article in the *Observer* (28 December 1986) entitled 'New Morality And The Sexual Time Bomb', writer Nicholas Wapshott is apparently concerned to distance himself from those who construct HIV/AIDS as a problem of and for homosexuality. He begins by announcing that 'AIDS is not the gay plague, nor ever was', and continues by discussing the risk to heterosexuals. However, this welcome tolerance and objectivity is exposed as a sham by his demand that we (and it is a 'we' which excludes lesbians and gay men by assumption) show 'sympathy and understanding for those [i.e. gay men] *trapped by their own proclivities*' (my emphasis). The *Concise Oxford Dictionary* defines 'proclivity' as 'Tendency to or towards object or habit, especially bad one', and the idea offered the reader is of gay men as helpless victims of (rather than as choosing, or having their lives enhanced by, or enjoying) their sexuality, and as such deserving of the sympathy and understanding commonly extended to 'victims' of other disasters or illnesses! Having denied the spurious link between AIDS and homosexuality, there is an immediate retrenchment; by characterizing AIDS as something affecting people who are the powerless victims of their bad sexual habits (homosexuality), Wapshott promptly recreates, in deceitfully liberal terms, the very association he purports to disavow.

Clearly it was not only the familiar bigotry of the tabloid press which set the agenda for the British response to the epidemic. The 'quality' newspapers, supposedly more intelligent, more liberal and tolerant, were just as ready to allocate blame.

Guilt by differentiation

It is the press who have created the widely accepted distinction between the 'innocent victims' of HIV/AIDS and those who, by that logic, are presumed 'guilty'. It is commonly asserted that haemophiliacs and others who became infected by the medical use of contaminated blood are 'innocent', as are babies and children infected either at birth or through medical procedures. All other infected individuals are deemed to have brought their suffering on themselves, usually through behaviour regarded as 'deviant': injecting drug use, homosexuality, prostitution and (less frequently) heterosexual promiscuity. Clearly the situation of an HIV+ baby or child is tragic. It would be monstrous to suggest otherwise. Yet all too often the press treatment of the stories of such children is manipulated in such a way as to suggest, at best, that the situation of HIV+ gay men, drug users or prostitutes is somehow less tragic, or at worst, that these groups are to be blamed, not only for their own illness but for the threat which they represent to the 'innocent'. It is quite illogical to blame people for behaviour which only *retrospectively* has been recognized as risky (since most people found to be HIV+ in the 1980s would probably have been infected before information about HIV transmission was available). It is also thoughtless and irresponsible to blame an entire group for the behaviour of some of its members. It is clearly ridiculous to include coffee drinkers or cigarette smokers in the category of 'at risk' drug users; similarly those gay men whose long term couple-relationships differ very little from what we think of as 'good marriages' cannot reasonably be regarded in the same light as the media stereotype of the 'promiscuous urban homosexual'. It is not who you are but what you do that puts you at risk, a simple fact which was not reflected in the AIDS reporting of the British press.

Thus *Woman's Own* (3 May 1986) reported the words of a mother whose baby was infected as a result of a transfusion: 'I've got nothing against the homosexual community ... but they were consenting adults, they *did* have a choice' (emphasis in original). In a similar vein, the *Sunday People* (3 November 1985) reports on the story of two children referred to in its headline as 'Innocent Victims Of The AIDS Scare'. '[N]ormally', the article tells us, 'the killer disease [sic] is transmitted by homosexuals or drug users. Little N and R just happen to have the blood complaint called haemophilia, some of whose sufferers have been infected with the AIDS antibodies.' A careful reading of the story reveals that the two children did *not* in fact have AIDS, nor were they even HIV+. The *Sunday People*'s interest in them was simply that the risk of contracting HIV has added to the anxiety of lives already complicated by haemophilia. Undoubtedly this is so, but it is equally true that, for example, gay men's lives, already complicated by the struggle to live in a deeply prejudiced society, have been burdened by the added fear of contracting HIV. Imagine the *Sunday People* publishing a similarly sympathetic piece about the plight of a gay man! A cynical reader, noting that the emphasis of the piece is on 'homosexuals or drug users' *transmitting* the 'killer disease', with no recognition of the fact that these groups, rather than being simply agents of infection, may be *affected* by HIV/AIDS, would be right in assuming that sympathy for either group is not on the *Sunday People*'s agenda.

The assertion that babies and children are innocent victims, while gay men, drug users and prostitutes 'have a choice', is a pervasive one. Clearly, informed and responsible behaviour is central to the prevention of HIV transmission. Yet to believe that avoiding HIV infection is at all times and in all places within the power of the individual is clearly nonsense. Given what is now known about the incubation period of HIV, it is probable that large numbers became infected (unsuspecting journalists perhaps among them) years before the virus or the illnesses associated with it were recognized. Equally, faced with a government prepared to prevent gay men having access to accurate safer sex information (see above, p. 22), it was simply not possible for anyone in the UK, gay or not, to learn about HIV or about how to prevent its transmission early in the epidemic. Drug users, another marginalized group, do not by and large choose, in any meaningful way, to become dependent on injectable drugs. (The difficulties involved in persuading intelligent people not to smoke and the struggle which confronts anyone who tries to quit smoking offer us an insight into the complexity of drug addiction!) Nor do they 'choose' to re-use or to share injecting equipment. The discrepancy in HIV+ statistics between the two drug-injecting populations of Edinburgh and Glasgow (which are comparable in size) is a clear indicator that the degree of 'choice' an individual has in relation to drug-related HIV risk is largely due to circumstances outside their control. In Glasgow, where there was official support, including police support, for needle exchange schemes, rates of HIV infection among drug users were much lower than in Edinburgh, where such schemes met with hostility. For an individual who may have been addicted to an illegal injectable drug for some time *before they were aware of the existence of HIV* the degree of 'choice' they may be able to exercise to protect themselves against infection is in fact dependent on very many circumstances quite outside their control.

To imply that certain groups of people may deliberately choose to put themselves at risk of HIV infection is outrageous. There is much justifiable sympathy expressed for the plight of haemophiliacs who, all unknowingly, became infected through contaminated Factor 8 (a blood-clotting protein obtained from donated blood). Clearly, there is no element of choice involved in whether or not to become haemophiliac. The question of how far being gay is a matter for choice is much debated, and there are some heterosexuals who believe that people whose sexual desire differs from their own are by definition blameworthy. Yet when considering the question of responsibility for becoming infected with HIV, there is no difference in 'innocence' between haemophiliacs and those gay men who unwittingly put themselves at risk because they had no information about HIV, its causes, or strategies for prevention. It is absurd to suggest that people should be held responsible for protecting themselves against something which was not known to exist, and to assert that such groups 'had a choice' is to impute to them nothing less than the gift of prophecy.

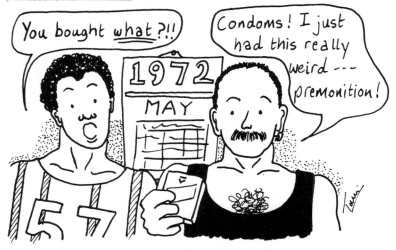

Of course, what is also being implied is that gay men and drug users do have a choice about whether or not to *be* gay men or drug users. They are not obliged, the argument goes, to have sex or to use drugs. What is at issue here is a naive and ill-informed set of beliefs about sex and drugs. Of course no-one is 'obliged' to take drugs, whether those drugs be nicotine, alcohol, caffeine or heroin, but the notion that simple, individual 'free choice' may be called into play and a logical decision made whether or not to begin using a particular drug is simply unsupportable. Drug use does not happen in a vacuum, as anyone who has tried to stop drinking or to give up coffee will understand. We live, all of us, in a drug-using culture, and we are, all of us, social beings. The social custom which dictates buying a round in a bar, offering someone a cigarette, or meeting a friend for coffee is no different in kind from that which dictates the use of marijuana or heroin in other circles. Such pressures are extremely powerful, and those who resist are seen as deviant.

Equally, the question of 'choice' is largely illusory in relation to sex. Research such as that carried out by the Women, Risk and AIDS Project based at Goldsmith's College in London, or by Nicola Gavey at the Psychology Department in the University of Auckland, has shown that women in general have very little choice in whether or not men will have sex with them. Men and women whose sexual relationships are based on negotiation and mutuality are still a privileged minority, and the ability to negotiate safe sex is far from the reality of most women's lives. Yet those who demand that gay men should not 'give in' to their desires for sex (for example, it is not uncommon for church leaders to say that it is fine to *be* gay, as long as you practise chastity and do not have sex) would be unlikely to accept that heterosexual men might justifiably be asked to do the same, despite evidence that such a move would have a much greater effect on the global epidemic of HIV/AIDS.

Blame, ignorance and the struggle to promote health

In the United States now, someone dies with AIDS every half an hour. This is in no sense an epidemic we can be sure of vanquishing. Professor Michael Adler, an HIV/AIDS specialist working at the Middlesex Hospital, points out in *AIDS Newsletter* that there is no sign of the rate of increase of infection slowing, and describes the overall prospect as 'very grim'. Until (or unless) a vaccine is developed and freely and cheaply available worldwide – something which has never happened in the history of scientific medicine – health promotion remains our only means of slowing the alarming spread of this particularly unpleasant virus. In a world where charitable organizations are forced to beg for donations in order to distribute the simple vaccine which would prevent millions of children dying from measles, the hope of bringing the HIV/AIDS epidemic under control with a vaccine seems, to say the least, remote. Health promotion is not a stop-gap measure until we can bring in the 'real' solution of scientific medicine; it will almost certainly remain the only practical strategy against HIV/AIDS for the foreseeable future.

In order for health promotion to be effective, an unprecedented process of education is needed for every individual on the planet. It is obvious that information is not, of itself, sufficient to result in global behaviour change, or the tobacco industry for one would have long ago ceased functioning. Yet without it, nobody will know either how or why behaviour change is needed. Only when *everyone* has accurate information about the virus, its transmission and how to protect themselves from infection will it be possible to slow the epidemic down.

The distortions, sensationalism and victimization which have characterized press coverage of the epidemic are in no sense harmless. On the simplest level, inaccuracy may lead to confusion, complacency or panic. On 8 September 1987, the *Guardian* stated that 'by the end of August 1,013 cases [of AIDS] had been reported, of whom 572 had died'. On the same day, the *Daily Star* told its readers that 'AIDS has now killed more than 1,000 people in Britain'. Which account is to be believed? At a time when a new virus, commonly deadly in its effects, is spreading at a steadily increasing rate among the population, surely simple accuracy is not too much to expect of our newspapers? Other implications of the media response to HIV/AIDS are, however, even more alarming, directly increasing the risk of harm to every section of their readership, whether lesbian, gay, heterosexual or bisexual.

Increasing the risk to lesbians and gay men

Firstly, there can be no doubt that press reporting of HIV/AIDS issues has commonly consisted of little more than incitement to hatred. That such reportage has very real consequences for people's behaviour may be seen by incidents early in 1985, following on the death with AIDS of a prison chaplain. Sensationalist reporting of this death, accompanied (as we have already seen) by alarmist fears about the possibility of infection via the communion chalice, resulted in ambulance workers, fire-fighters and First Aid staff declaring that they would not rescue gay men in emergency situations; and even now, ambulance workers in some divisions carry resuscitation devices as protection against the imagined 'risk' of contracting HIV during mouth-to-mouth resuscitation, despite the fact that such devices may impede rather than expedite the saving of lives.

Ambulance workers, fire-fighters and First Aiders are not by and large considered to be among the more hysterical and panic-stricken members of the population. Yet the 'risk' of becoming HIV+ by rescuing an infected individual from a burning building, giving them mouth-to-mouth resuscitation, or even treating a freely bleeding wound is so remote as to be beyond the bounds of necessary consideration, a fact which the workers in question must have been well aware of. Their refusal to render assistance to gay men, far from representing an illogical overreaction to such a minuscule threat, must be seen as the only rational response to the veritable tidal wave of panic-mongering to which they had been subjected by the press. In the face of this tide of misinformation (published, of course, for profit, and therefore restricted neither by respect for the truth nor by responsibility for the public health), the reassurances of health promoters (published, of course, at public expense, and therefore restricted by tight budgets and official moralism) are reduced to a tiny, unheeded whisper. A brief anecdote from personal experience serves to illustrate the effectiveness of this panic-mongering.

Going to help at the scene of a road accident in May 1990, I saw a young woman lying in the road surrounded by a small crowd. She had been knocked down by a cyclist, who, as might have been expected, was standing in a daze, staring at the steadily growing pool of blood on the tarmac by her head. It was less easy to understand why everyone else was behaving in the same scared way, standing some distance away, simply staring. It was only when I bent down to talk to the woman that the mystery was solved. 'Don't touch her!', came a breathless cry. 'You might get AIDS!' The implications of this still horrify me. Have we been so bamboozled by sensationalist reporting that we are prepared to let someone bleed to death rather than risk 'catching AIDS'? This woman was not self-evidently a member of one of the supposed 'risk groups' so misleadingly created by epidemiologists. She was neither Black nor a gay man, and she certainly did not look like the stereotype of a prostitute or an 'addict'. Yet the hysteria of HIV/AIDS reportage had directly put her life at risk, as it puts all our lives at risk. It has so stigmatized and sensationalized 'AIDS' that she might have bled to death in the middle of the road while the onlookers stood, paralysed with a quite irrational fear.

What would have happened if she had been an obviously gay man is, of course, open to conjecture merely. However, the press have not been content simply to spread lies about the risk of contracting HIV by reckless contact with chalices or homosexuals. There have been frequent and quite astonishing calls for direct violence to be directed against *all* gay men. In 1986, the *Daily Express* ranted that 'The homosexuals who have brought this plague upon us should be locked up. Burning is too good for them. Bury them in a pit and pour on quicklime', while in December of the same year, one Councillor Brownhill, leader of South Staffordshire Council, was widely reported as demanding that 90 per cent of gay men should be 'exterminated in gas chambers' in order to tackle the 'AIDS crisis'. Such remarks, if directed at groups protected (however inadequately) by legislation, such as those from minority ethnic groups, would be punishable by law. No such legislation exists to protect lesbians and gays, and the *Daily Express* is quite free to demand that they should be buried alive in quicklime. These obscene sentiments do not only appeal to a violent minority. I have frequently heard otherwise charming and reasonable young people around the country regurgitate similar sentiments, insisting that the only way of beating the epidemic is to 'put all the queers on an island', 'put them against a wall and shoot them', 'lock them all up in concentration camps' (yes, really) or 'castrate them all'. Do we really want our young people growing up in a culture where heterosexuality is characterized by such empty-headed viciousness?

Such virulent and freely expressed hatred is obviously dangerous to lesbians and gay men. LESPOP, the London organization which monitors attacks on lesbians and gay men in co-operation with the police, believes that the link between AIDS and homosexuality fostered by the press has resulted in increased attacks on lesbians and gay men, attacks which sometimes result in their murder. It is a particularly appalling burden for young gay men and lesbians, who, already obliged to struggle for recognition of their sexuality with precious little support (and that little steadily being eroded as a result of prejudiced legislation such as Section 28 of the 1988 Local Government Act – see p. 107), are now forced to realize that they have to struggle for recognition of their very right to life itself. There are more lesbians and gay men in Britain than there are bus drivers or teachers; the cost in terms of human suffering, stress and misery is considerable. It is unsurprising, though it is a cause for national shame, that very many of our young lesbians and gay men attempt suicide. The extraordinarily powerful nature of the stigma attached to homosexuality is revealed in the insolent and disgusting treatment meted out to the Princess of Wales when she was brave enough to visit publicly the bedside of a personal friend dying with AIDS, a gay man. What can she be thinking of, thundered the *Sun*'s Gary Bushell: 'Does she want to be known as the patron saint of sodomy?' That such vitriol can be directed at so popular a national icon as Princess Di is some indication of the deep-rootedness of the hatred and revulsion expressed towards homosexuality by the British press. It takes something pretty remarkable to sully the universal adoration with which the Princess of Wales is generally regarded.

It is important to recognize that the hostile homophobia of the British gutter press is not the only possible response to the HIV/ AIDS epidemic. In the USA, for example, Emmanuel Dreuilhe writes in *Mortal Embrace*, his autobiographical account of his battle with AIDS, 'I now know that English AIDS patients must suffer not only assaults from the virus but also the attacks of Fleet Street, those tabloids that go after the victims instead of the epidemic.' He writes with some amazement of 'the shame of English AIDS victims', and comments sadly, 'How heavily English homophobia must weigh on

[them]!' Although anti-gay bigotry is the norm rather than the exception in most countries in the world, the particular nastiness of the British tabloid press has a character all its own.

Increasing the risk to heterosexuals

The increased risk to heterosexuals which is a direct consequence of inaccurate and sensational press coverage of HIV/AIDS is twofold. Firstly, as we have seen, a public convinced that you can 'catch AIDS' from all manner of casual contact is liable to leave any one of us who has an accident bleeding in the gutter or suffocating to death. Secondly, the relentless insistence that AIDS is not a heterosexual problem leaves the majority of the population unforgivably vulnerable to infection. Homophobia has always been dangerous for homosexuals; it is now potentially deadly for heterosexuals.

An article appearing in the *Sun* early in 1990 (in response to the death of actor Ian Charleson with AIDS) is typical of this deadly trend. Fiona Macdonal Hull, writing, it must be remembered, in a year when there was a *doubling* of reported heterosexual cases of AIDS, vehemently denies any connection between AIDS and heterosexuals, and launches a vigorous attack on 'homosexuals' (gender, as usual, unspecified). Claiming that Ian Charleson died because he 'caught AIDS' (sic), she demands that 'Our gay community [must] face up to the fact that AIDS is a homosexual, drug-related disease. It is not a heterosexual disease. It becomes a heterosexual disease *only* when gays or drug addicts become either blood donors or switch sides. It is time the homosexuals and drug addicts cleaned up their act. They, and they alone, are responsible for people dying from AIDS.'

Here we recognize the familiar twisted logic which asserts that groups affected by HIV are somehow responsible for it. Yet no newspaper has, for example, claimed that young women who use tampons are 'responsible for people dying from toxic shock syndrome' (interestingly the press have shown themselves quite capable of differentiating between a 'syndrome' and a 'disease' in the case of toxic shock, as they seem quite unable to do in relation to AIDS), nor have there been any calls for the criminalization of members of the American Legion for 'being responsible' for Legionnaires' Disease. In what way, one wonders, may 'homosexuals and drug addicts' be said to be 'responsible' for HIV; are they supposed to have developed it in secret laboratories? The equally familiar rhetoric of exclusion now excludes both 'homosexuals' and 'drug addicts' from the category 'people'; there is no sense in which these two despised groups are identified as deserving of support because *they* are 'dying from AIDS'. Interestingly, 'drug addicts' are, in this piece, similarly excluded from the category 'heterosexuals'. That piece of nonsense is quite in line with the notion that a disease, being either heterosexual or homosexual, is somehow capable of having a sexual identity!

In addition to the wilful sacrifice of logic to prejudice, this short piece contains enough straightforward medical misinformation to undo in one fell swoop years of careful health education. AIDS is described as 'a disease', and as something one can catch, when in fact it is a syndrome and impossible either to catch or to transmit. It is also described as 'a homosexual disease', as though it were possible for a virus (which has no gender and does not have any variety of sex) to be either (a) associated exclusively with a particular sexual identity or (b) capable of recognizing the sexual identity of its 'proper' victims. In addition, the assertion that AIDS is a 'homosexual, drug-related disease' is thoroughly confused and confusing. Are there no heterosexual drug users? Do only homosexual drug users get AIDS? If so, then heterosexual drug users and non-drug-using homosexuals presumably are not at risk. If it is 'drug-related', what drug(s) are we talking about? Paracetamol? Alcohol? Marijuana? And in what way is 'AIDS' drug-related? It is of course quite misleading to describe AIDS as drug-related (except in so far as drug therapies are usually used in the treatment of opportunistic infections), and simply inadequate to associate HIV infection with drug use. HIV transmission between drug users may only occur if injecting equipment used by an already infected individual is immediately used by a non-infected individual without appropriate cleaning in between users. This is a simple and straightforward piece of information, analogous perhaps to our understanding that it is not advisable to share someone's snotty handkerchief if you do not want to catch their cold. Yet few would describe the common cold as 'cotton-linked'.

Perhaps the most disturbing characteristic of this piece is its hysterical refutation of the possibility of 'heterosexual AIDS'. Heterosexual infection is put down to gays or drug addicts becoming blood donors or 'switching sides', as though heterosexuality and homosexuality were opposing armies in some bizarre war game (which, clearly, to Fiona Macdonal Hull, they are). Here yet again is that most irresponsible and deadly lie of the tabloid press, that AIDS is somehow intrinsic to homosexuality, and that heterosexuals need only to protect themselves from homosexuality in order to protect themselves from AIDS. To ignore completely the vast numbers of heterosexuals ill or dying with AIDS around the world, in order to manufacture false evidence against the hated homosexuals of one's own small country, is deeply insulting to those heterosexuals and to their families. Clearly, 'foreign' heterosexuals may be written off with as much impunity as home-grown homosexuals. The implication that a heterosexual could *only* become infected by HIV by means of donated blood infected by homosexuals or drug users, or by having sex with a homosexual (or a drug user?) who had 'changed sides' (and exactly how does a drug user change sides?), is potentially lethal for heterosexuals. Given its professed hatred of homosexuality you would expect the tabloid press to do everything within its power to enable its heterosexual readers (and it is abundantly clear that the tabloids do not believe that any other sort exists) to protect themselves from infection with the 'killer disease'.

It is this contradiction at the heart of the AIDS reporting of the tabloid press which reveals the true nature of the beast. The responsibility to their heterosexual readers, who need clear information and a realistic perception of their own level of risk if they are to survive, is secondary to the need to whip up hatred against gay men. What we are witnessing here is categorically *not* an attempt to defend heterosexuals against an epidemic infection. It is, rather, a desperate attempt to defend heterosexuality against homosexuality, and as such, belongs to the threatened, anxious and punitive ideology of the moral right.

The beast from the closet: threatened norms

There are competing explanations as to why the monogamous, heterosexual, nuclear family unit has such a uniquely powerful place in political life, and why any supposed 'threat to the family' is met with such outrage and indignation. After all, the 'traditional' family of dad, mum, two kids and perhaps a golden labrador is now the living situation of only a minority, and can no longer be thought of as the norm. Yet it is still thought of as norm*al*, despite increasing recognition of social realities such as high divorce rates, wife-beating and the widespread neglect and abuse of children (physical, mental and sexual). Moreover, it is frequently claimed that a secure social order depends upon the preservation of the family. Why is the family accorded such importance?

Traditionally, Marxism has answered by pointing to the Industrial Revolution, when the split between a public life of paid labour and a private life of restful, leisured domesticity created the family as we think of it today. The family unit, Marxists have argued, is essential to capitalism. The unpaid labour of women in the home has ensured the reproduction of the future labour force, while maintaining the current labour force well fed, well cared for, healthy and sexually serviced. In addition, by 'the worker' being constructed as male and as head of a household, entitled to a 'family wage', women have been made available as a 'reserve army of labour', willing because of their domestic responsibilities to work part-time for low pay; an army which capital is then free to recruit to and reject from the labour market as fluctuating economic conditions dictate.

Feminism, on the other hand, has identified the role of the family in ensuring women's continued subordination to men. Conditioned to see their highest duty in life as that of wife and mother, content to find their own fulfilment in wifely devotion and care for their children, women are unable to compete with men in education, career or politics. Indeed, their subordinate position in the home, literally as the possession of one man or another (first father, then husband, finally, in widowhood, son), was until recently reinforced in law (and indeed still is in many cultures).

Whether the politics behind the drive to defend the nuclear family be sexual or economic, or both, it plays a key role in all conservative ideologies, where its power is rendered absolute by appeals to its status as 'natural'. There are of course an almost infinite number of possible kinship structures, and a brief glance at history, or at other cultures, reveals as wishful thinking the suggestion that our particular notion of the family is 'natural'. Yet ideas of 'naturalness' exert a powerful appeal in a post-modern world suspicious of the artificial and well aware of the dangers of the Faustian bargain of technological supremacy. It is perhaps unsurprising that AIDS has been interpreted by many as another of a long list of evils, from cancer to global warming, blamed on 'going against nature'. This interpretation depends, of course, on ignoring the heterosexual majority of people with HIV/AIDS, since it is homosexuality, not heterosexuality, which is widely perceived as 'unnatural'. Indeed, 'unnatural acts' is a familiar euphemism for homosexual activity. Animals, we are assured, would not do such things. In fact, homosexual acts (and, in some species, homosexual *preference*) exist widely among animals, birds, fish and insects, being probably no more unusual in the animal kingdom than monogamous pairing for life. An interesting comparison may be drawn with rape which, although it is almost unknown among animals, is most certainly not characterized as 'unnatural' when carried out by humans. Indeed, some excuse rape on the grounds of a man's 'natural' irrepressible sex drive or innate aggression.

Can sex be called 'natural' at all? Social scientists on the whole agree that such an idea is fairly meaningless. Human sexual behaviour is learned, social behaviour. It is among the most ritualized, politicized and artificial of human behaviours, and everywhere subject to legislative and societal controls and strictures. Yet we stubbornly cling to the idea that the 'right' and 'wrong' ways of having sex, which have been imposed on us by our particular socialization in our particular culture at our particular historical time, are deeply rooted in nature. Interwoven with such beliefs is the idea of going against not only nature, but god.

Any challenge to the naturalness of family life is frequently met by appeals to the codes of religion, sets of strictures and narratives which are believed to stretch back before humanity, and to overarch mere history or anthropology. Those extremely powerful bodies, the churches, line up in defence of the family as natural, necessary, ordained by god, a 'Holy Family'. The almighty, the supernatural, is of course a trump card against the dissatisfaction expressed by Marxists, feminists etc., since the argument is promptly taken out of the realm of logic and the demonstrable, and into the realm of mysticism and the supernatural. God intended men and women to have sex only in order to propagate, and only within the bound of holy matrimony – end of argument. It is equally impossible to argue with US Congressman William Dannemeyer's fatuous observation that 'God's plan for man [sic] was Adam and Eve and not Adam and Steve', a statement routinely trotted out by religious fundamentalists as though it represented unequivocal truth. However laughable moral majority representatives such as American televangelist Jerry Falwell or our own ex-Chief Inspector of Police James Anderton may seem when they insist that AIDS is divine retribution, they have a powerful hold on the imagination of many people. Such beliefs cannot but have a very real influence on the course of the epidemic, whether by allowing 'the just' to neglect precautions against HIV infection, by encouraging abusive and oppressive treatment of those already infected, or by forbidding the dissemination of accurate and explicit information to all who need it. It is alarmingly clear that social policy decisions about everything from public education to care of people with HIV/AIDS are open to manipulation by vociferous lobby groups motivated by punitive fundamentalism. But is there any truth in what they say?

Sex and drugs and retribution: the truth

Faced with the assertion that AIDS is somehow a punishment for sin, many people find it hard to resist uneasy agreement. After all, the 'risk groups' are by and large social deviants, are they not? It is unarguably the case that the *majority* of people known to have HIV or AIDS in Britain are gay men, and that injecting drug users too represent a sizeable number of those affected. So is there not, after all, a grain of truth in the idea that it was the 'bad behaviour' of such

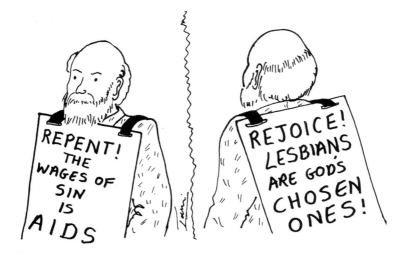

people that put them at risk? Perhaps, as we have heard from mosque, synagogue, temple and church, AIDS is the just deserts of sinners?

The key question in this debate is that of identities versus acts. In Rabbi Julia Neuberger's much-quoted observation, it is a strange god indeed who punishes male homosexuals but seems to protect female homosexuals; who strikes down those who inject drugs while withholding his wrath from those who sniff, smoke or swallow them. One could go further; if we are trying to read a message from the divinity in the smoking entrails of epidemiology, then we must deduce that lesbians, among whom the sexual trans-mission of HIV is very rare, are the chosen ones. There has been conspicuous silence from mullah, pontiff and archbishop alike on that point.

The fundamental 'truth' about HIV/AIDS is simply that it is *not* who you are that matters, it is *what you do*. It is quite possible to be a life-long drug user or even an addict without in any way increasing your likelihood of becoming HIV+. Smoking, sniffing or swallow-ing any drug, whether it be nicotine, marijuana, cocaine, heroin, amphetamine or whatever, will decidedly not involve any risk of HIV infection. Nor, indeed, will injecting a drug. It is merely the act of *sharing injecting equipment* which involves risk. And if the act of sharing drug-using equipment is sinful, perhaps we should consider questioning the habit of passing alcohol among Christian congregations in a shared chalice?

The question of sexual sin is similarly specific. Certain sexual *acts* have the potential to transmit HIV, others do not. A promiscuous gay man who practises safe sex is unlikely to become infected. The pre-eminent sexual practice for the transmission of HIV is anal intercourse, a practice which is widely identified in the public mind with gay men. Yet studies (such as those published by the British long-term study of gay men's sexual practices, Project Sigma) have quite conclusively shown that there are many gay men who seldom or never have sex in this way, while according to such well-known classics of sex research as *The Hite Report*, many heterosexual couples do. Sex manuals aimed at the heterosexual market, such as Alex Comfort's well-known *Joy of Sex*, routinely include advice about anal intercourse. Similarly, lesbians are not at low risk for HIV because god loves lesbians more than heterosexual women, but because their sexual practices are largely 'safe'. Lesbians have always been noted for a remarkably low rate of STD (sexually transmitted disease) infection generally, and lesbians are more at risk from HIV through practices such as unsafe drug use or unprotected sex with men than from 'deviant' sex with each other.

Clearly, if we are inclined to interpret HIV as punishment, then it is neither illegal drug use nor sexual 'deviance' which is being punished. Yet the strongest argument against the divine retributionists remains the indisputable fact that they are simply ignoring the millions of people infected through 'normal' heterosexual sex, and ensuring by their warped message that many thousands more will become infected, believing themselves to be not at risk.

AIDS in the service of social control

When the only 'legitimate' sexuality is the punitively narrow one of the penetration of a woman's vagina by the penis of her legally married husband, the very existence of lesbians and gay men is anathema. And when lesbians and gay men begin asserting, as they have over the last twenty years, that their lives are capable of as much richness, happiness and love as anyone else's, that assertion is intolerable. Worse, when feminists insist, as they do, that lesbians (and by implication, gay men) are not born but made, that any woman is capable of becoming a lesbian, and that for many women it is the best option, politically, sexually and emotionally, such pronouncements are heresy. The homosexual is identified as posing a threat to the sanctity of the family, so if it is true that anyone could be 'recruited' to the ranks of the homosexual, then it must be made impossible for anyone in their right mind to want to do so. In other words, homosexuality must be stigmatized to such an extent that the social punishment it attracts makes it an unimaginable option for anyone considering 'changing sides'.

This is the explanation of the strategy of exclusion which we have seen operating in the AIDS reportage of the tabloid press. Homosexuals are symbolically cast out of the 'public', out of 'normal communion', finally out of the category of 'people' or 'the human race' itself. The message is clear: homosexuality is itself a terrible fate, and is itself contaminating, diseased, dangerous. How impossible it would be, then, for the tabloids to avoid blurring the distinction between AIDS and homosexuality itself, to such a degree that we may read of 'AIDS suspects', as though being ill was a criminal offence. To be suspected of having this 'disease', which has been so thoroughly linked with homosexuality, is to lose all right to respect, privacy or honour, no matter what the circumstances. Thus, as Simon Watney points out in his book *Policing Desire*, the story of a man who died rescuing others in the King's Cross underground fire could be reported as 'Blaze Hero In AIDS Scare', and the dead man dismissed as a 'deadly AIDS carrier'. This is why the press, having set up the association between homosexuality and AIDS in the mind of its (heterosexual) readers, must present any story which does not fit the pattern as an exception which proves the rule.

Thus *Woman's Own* tells us (12 July 1986) 'The Sad, Sad Story Of The Woman With AIDS', the case of a woman who contracted HIV through heterosexual sex and is now seriously ill with AIDS. 'No-one told her', we read, 'that sleeping with a man could be like facing a firing squad ... no-one said that sex – normal, healthy, conventional sex – could kill.' The hidden message here is of course that it is obvious that the 'other' kind of sex, for which read *ab*normal, *un*healthy, *un*conventional gay sex, can kill. We are invited to be as surprised as the central figure that 'normal' sex can kill, that sex characterized as 'healthy' can in fact be just as unhealthy as 'abnormal' sex. We are to interpret this case as the exception which proves the rule.

As the spurious link between homosexuality and AIDS is strengthened, so too vicious expressions of hatred and the desire to punish people with AIDS themselves become commonplace. The *News of the World* (1 March 1986) reports the results of a poll of its readers, 56.8 per cent of whom were in favour of the suggestion that 'AIDS carriers [sic] should be sterilised and given treatment to curb their sexual appetite.' The *same poll*, clearly reinforcing the link between sexual identity and AIDS, questioned readers about their attitudes to homosexuality, and 57 per cent were reported to be in favour of its recriminalization. When we consider the fact that people infected with HIV (whom the article misleadingly refers to as 'AIDS carriers') may be newborn babies, pregnant women or the elderly and infirm, and that it makes no sense whatever to call for the sterilization of such groups, or for 'treatment to curb their sexual appetite', it becomes glaringly obvious that 'AIDS carrier' is taken to mean *homosexual*. Nowhere is the grotesque cruelty of urging the sterilization, drugging, quarantining, imprisoning or castration of people ill with a frightening and ghastly condition questioned, though the papers in which such sentiments are promulgated are often precisely those that boast of their readers' heartwarming generosity in supporting a variety of sponsored charitable stunts.

Later on in the epidemic, the link between homosexuality and AIDS is now being defended more overtly. We are familiar with press reports insisting that we have 'overreacted' to 'the AIDS scare', and more responsible journalists now take time to criticize their less thoughtful colleagues for taking this line. Thus Lynn Barber, writing in the *Independent on Sunday* (8 March 1992), takes Richard Ingrams to task for an article in the second issue of his magazine *The Oldie*, in which he asserts that there is no heterosexual risk and that 'homosexuals only want us to believe there is because otherwise we would be prejudiced against them for spreading disease'. Barber calls his argument 'bizarre' and 'addled', and refers to Ingrams' homophobia as 'wicked', but the fact remains that what Ingrams is doing is publicly protecting and reinforcing the tired old link between homosexuals and AIDS. The very terms of the current argument were set in the early years of the epidemic by the homophobia of the British press, and the legacy of that is still very much with us.

Death by misinformation

The article in *Woman's Own* lamented the fact that 'nobody had told' the woman concerned about the possibility of contracting HIV heterosexually. The real tragedy, of course, is that there has never been a shortage of people desperate to tell her just that. It is the mythology of AIDS created by a press obsessively concerned with its own nasty brand of 'queer-bashing' which aided and abetted the ignorance which led to her illness.

If the press shows no regard for the need for accuracy in the cause of fighting the epidemic, it shows less than none for the needs or feelings of those already infected. Thus, the *Woman's Own* article continues in this vein: 'Nor did they tell her that it would be a slow and painful end, filled with suffering, almost constant agony and illness. That she would enter a twilight world from which death, when it came, would be a welcome relief.' This is, as we have seen, a very simplistic, one-sided account of what it may be like to have AIDS. Nowhere do we find mention of the thousands of people living with AIDS for whom life is still full, still satisfying, still joyful. It is painful to imagine the feelings of someone who had just been diagnosed HIV+ reading that account.

Health professionals are deeply worried by the widespread failure of heterosexuals to take HIV seriously, demonstrated by survey after survey showing that condom use is sporadic at best and still not seen as necessary by many. It is not that they do not have the information; most people are, on the whole, remarkably well informed about HIV and AIDS, and know how to protect themselves. Yet people seem to be refusing to recognize that they need to do so. With the vitriolic outpourings of our national press insisting that AIDS equals homosexuality equals something disgusting that 'normal' people should not have to worry about, it is hardly surprising that there is such an entrenched resistance to the idea of heterosexual risk.

This resistance is both expressed and reinforced by press coverage later on in the epidemic. The *Telegraph* for example, which on 2 May 1983 was depicting AIDS in dramatic headlines as 'Wages of Sin: A Deadly Toll', was by 5 June 1988 insisting that there was *no risk* to heterosexuals, and that the notion of heterosexual spread had been propagated by a 'gay conspiracy'. The *Sunday Times* (5 June 1988) echoed this, speaking of the 'myth of heterosexual spread'. This wilful refusal to understand that more people have become infected with HIV through heterosexual sex than through any other means can only be understood in the context of an imperative need to vilify the idea of homosexuality and to protect the idea of heterosexuality from contamination by the idea of a disease linked with deviant sex. Ironically, of course, it is the one approach which is most likely to result in real heterosexuals being infected with a real virus. The virus, unlike British journalism, cannot discriminate between social groups and entirely lacks that sense of moral outrage which might lead it to target the stigmatized and vilified.

The interests of heterosexuals have not been well served by the anti-gay approach of the press. More worryingly still, there is plenty of evidence, both in the USA and in Britain, that social policy makers allowed the epidemic to get a hold *because they believed that it 'only' affected gay men*. Even now, official statements to the effect that 'AIDS is not *only* a gay problem' suggest that gays are not worth worrying about. Health workers at New York City Hospital dubbed AIDS 'Wrath of God Syndrome' (the acronym, WOGS, managing to be doubly offensive) in the early days of the epidemic, a bitter revelation of the entrenched homophobia which has left us all, lesbian, gay, heterosexual or bisexual, with an appalling health crisis. The lesbian and gay community has responded by taking action to protect its members and to educate and inform everybody. Heterosexuals who are lulled into smugness by their own homophobia and that of the press are left ill equipped to deal with this epidemic. It is not ignorance which is killing people, it is deliberate misinformation in the service of bigotry.

3

Weaker vessels: HIV/AIDS and women

HIV/AIDS does not exist in a vacuum. Indeed, as we have already seen, the course of the epidemic must be considered in relation to already existing social patterns, prejudices and power struggles. HIV does have specific medical implications for women's health – for example, human papilloma virus (which causes cervical cancer) is much more invasive in women who have AIDS – but the particular situation of women in this epidemic can only be understood in the wider context of their position in society, and in particular in the context of their relationship to the scientific and medical communities.

There exists a large and authoritative body of feminist research (including the work of Barbara Ehrenreich, Dierdre English, Lesley Doyal, Renate D. Klein, Ann Oakley, Hilary Homans, Sophie Laws, Diana Scully and Pauline Bart, to name but a few) which indicates that women's position *vis-à-vis* the health care system is fundamentally different from that of men in several important ways, all of which have a bearing on their experiences as people affected by HIV/AIDS. Firstly, women are overwhelmingly the providers of health care in our society, a pattern which is repeated around the world. The NHS in Britain has a workforce which is 75 per cent female; it is still the case that the vast majority of nurses are women, as are most health visitors. Yet women are, throughout the NHS, in lower-paid, lower-status jobs than men, and are grossly underrepresented in the decision-making bodies which govern the service. At a more basic level, primary health care is provided by women on an informal (and largely unrecognized) basis day to day.

It is almost exclusively women who are personally responsible for maintaining the health of the family, a fact clearly recognized by the advertisers who promote 'healthy' foods such as low-fat margarines at housewives by playing on their concern for their husbands' and children's health. (Low-fat food aimed at women for their own consumption is, in contrast, sold on the premise that it will make them more attractive to men.) It is women who take children to the dentist, the optician or the clinic for their check-ups and vaccinations, women who take time off work to care for sick children, women who look after their sick male partners, women who care for elderly or disabled relatives. Additionally, women make up the greater part of the volunteer workforce providing a variety of services from meals on wheels to WRVS shops and other services in hospitals. Even at the Terrence Higgins Trust, Britain's most important AIDS service organization, over half the volunteers are women, despite the facts that the majority of the HIV+ clients served by the Trust are men and that the Trust has its roots in the gay male community.

A second important difference between women's relationship to health care and men's lies in the way in which the two sexes are regarded by the medical profession. Medical textbooks depict the male body as the norm, while referring to women's bodies as

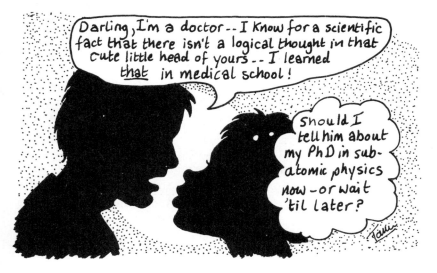

anything from a complicated, troublesome variation on the norm to an innately pathological entity. Additionally, women are believed to be intrinsically mentally unstable, a cultural stereotype which is both shared and reinforced by the medical profession. As recently as 1979, Karen Armitage carried out a comparative study (reported in Peter Aggleton's book *Health*, among others) of the behaviour of (male) doctors when consulted about a range of complaints such as fatigue, dizziness and headaches. Women who presented themselves as having such complaints were more likely to receive a *psychological* diagnosis, while their male counterparts were given more thorough *physical* examinations in an attempt to isolate a physiological cause for their symptoms. Men seem to be regarded within medicine as intrinsically more honest, more reliable, more stable and more likely to have 'real' health problems than women. Men's health also seems to be seen as simply more important, a straightforward reflection of their higher status within society. One result of this attitude is that women's health is a low priority for the health profession generally. Research into women's health issues is poorly funded, with the result that many conditions common to women are little understood and often misdiagnosed. The Endometriosis Society reports, for example, that it is common for women suffering from this painful condition (in which the lining of the womb grows in the abdominal cavity outside the womb, causing scarring and adhesions as a result of cyclical bleeding) to be dismissed as neurotic by their GPs and prescribed tranquillizers rather than given a thorough physical examination. Lack of empirical research on women's health makes it all too easy for poorly understood or unrecognized physiological problems to be attributed to neurosis. Work in the area of women's health is poorly esteemed, with concomitant low status for those who choose to do such work.

Thirdly, there has been a long process of medicalization of reproduction, by which, historically, control of the process of childbirth was wrested from the hands of (female) midwives into those of (male) obstetricians, and control of contraceptive and abortifacient remedies removed from the traditional female healers and restricted to the domain of scientific medicine. This has meant that women have come to represent a section of the population most accessible to medical scrutiny, obliged to attend hospital regularly on an out-patient basis during every pregnancy and to consult medical practitioners for contraception, abortion and related issues. Thus, by defining the biological processes of the female lifecycle as falling within the sphere of medicine, it becomes well nigh impossible for a woman to make it from the cradle to the grave without becoming a patient. It is medical practitioners too who make the decision as to who has an abortion and who is denied one, who is granted sterilization, who refused it and who dragooned into it, who is allowed contraceptive advice and supplies and who forbidden either, who is assisted in conceiving a child and who hindered, who is given drugs for menstrual pain and who given psychiatric treatment. This clearly gives rise to a very specific relationship between a woman and her own body, and between women and medicine. Women are accustomed both to being 'patients' and to being told their ailments are 'natural' or trivial or all in the mind. Additionally, the thousands of pregnant women attending antenatal clinics at any one time are a readily available population sample, a potential experimental group, which is obliging enough to come to the researcher, thus enabling the usual time-consuming process of selection and recruitment to be side-stepped (see p. 57).

Another important way in which the medical profession exercises control over women is by its jurisdiction over the field of sexuality. As the power of the pulpit gave way to the power of the microscope and scalpel, sexual behaviour was categorized no longer as a sin, but as a component of bodily health and, as such, open to regulation by the physician. Both men's and women's sexuality have been defined in a thoroughly distorted way by the medical profession. Men are 'naturally' supposed to be possessed of a virtually uncontrollable sexual 'drive', needing regular outlet for good health, while women are similarly defined as innately lacking in sexual desire, motivated instead by a longing for babies and a deep emotional need to serve men. One implication of this construction is that women are required to take responsibility for the sexual health of men, as they are for their general health, by making themselves available to relieve the 'sexual tension' of their mate, and by protecting him from anything which might arouse his sexual anxiety and lead him to impotence. (The staying power of this particular message may be deduced from the popular reference to demanding or successful women as 'castrating bitches'!) Additionally, 'healthy' sex has been exclusively defined as penis-in-vagina intercourse, a restriction which has tremendous implications for women's health. As feminist writer Sheila Jeffreys points out in her book *Anticlimax*, not only does such a narrow definition pathologize as 'deviant' any sexual coupling which does not involve a penis and a vagina (such as gay or lesbian sex), but it gives rise to a whole new set of 'medical' problems, such as vaginismus and 'premature' ejaculation. Such experiences can only be defined as problems if there is some kind of obligation to achieve penile penetration, and once they are defined as medical problems, in need of a medical solution, they act quite powerfully to reinforce the idea that sexual behaviour is the rightful province of doctors. In addition, placing such emphasis on penile penetration further emphasizes male orgasm and pleasure, while relegating female pleasure (located in the clitoris rather than the vagina) to a mere side effect of the process. It also requires women to depend upon chemical or mechanical forms of contraception to protect them from pregnancy, rather than seeking mutual pleasure in alternatives to penetrative sex.

If women are seen in medical eyes as subservient to the needs of men, they are seen as even more secondary to the needs of their children. In marriage, the physical and mental health of a woman is widely supposed by the medical profession to depend on her ability to conceive and bear children, while in pregnancy she is regarded as little more than a life-support system for the foetus. Anti-abortion campaigners and those who would withhold donor insemination from single women and lesbians are clear indicators of the widespread popular sentiment that women simply do not have the basic right to decide whether or not to have a child, a set of beliefs in clear conflict with the idea that it is in motherhood that a woman's primary fulfilment lies. Once she has given birth, the mother is blamed for almost everything which may befall her child subsequently, from bed-wetting to glue-sniffing, from homosexuality (she was an overprotective mother) to becoming a mass murderer (the mother of Peter Sutcliffe, the 'Yorkshire Ripper', was widely held to be responsible for his slaughtering women).

A rich vein of fear and loathing has always run through the Judaeo-Christian response to female sexuality from Genesis to St Paul (it runs through many other religions too, of course, but there is no space here to debate them all). Science has been dominated by men for centuries, and scientific objectivity has proved no match for misogyny. Doctors have joined with men of religion in firmly associating women's sexuality with contamination and disease. In the context of sexually transmitted diseases, women, especially prostitute women, have traditionally been seen as representing an active threat of infection to men, rather than as at risk from the illness themselves. Thus, when the great epidemics of syphilis swept across continents, popular engravings showed attractive women hiding death's-head grins behind masks. One such showed the 'head of a prostitute' who had died of syphilis. The head, half eaten away by disease and grossly disfigured, was presented not in order to evoke sympathy for the dead woman, but in order to arouse terror and loathing in the men who were understood to be her potential 'victims'. Such woman-blaming is not simply an excess of the distant past. As recently as the Second World War, public health campaigns focusing on syphilis and gonorrhoea relied heavily on images of seductive young women luring innocent men to their destruction, a theme as old as Circe, as modern as *Fatal Attraction.*

Women, then, are both disadvantaged and exploited by scientific medicine. Although comprising the bulk of the labour force in the formal health care sector, women are poorly paid and badly represented in the more prestigious and powerful health service jobs. They provide a vast network of informal health care entirely unpaid and mostly unrecognized, and in addition make up the majority of formal voluntary health care provision. Yet medicine serves their needs poorly, and functions, indeed, as a mechanism for maintaining their subordination to men.

Fitting AIDS in

So how does HIV/AIDS fit into this picture? Their second-class social status has clear implications for women affected by HIV/

AIDS, whether directly or indirectly. Clearly, women are responsible for most of the caring for people who are ill as a result of HIV/AIDS. There are, of course, large numbers of gay men involved in caring for these people, whether on a one-to-one basis of lover caring for lover, or as part of the network of 'buddies' which has evolved in many countries in the developed world to offer voluntary companionship and practical support to people sick with HIV-related illness. However, this has not altered the gender imbalance in the formal health care sector, and it is still largely women who, as mothers, partners or sisters, are taking on the burden of caring for family members ill with HIV disease. There are also large numbers of women, both lesbian and heterosexual, involved in the voluntary organizations which provide care and support for people affected by HIV/AIDS, and it is usually the mother, often ill herself, who has to care for a child born with HIV infection.

The long-standing view of women as innately contaminating and diseased has echoed through what has been said or written about AIDS. Thus we find women referred to in many medical writings as 'vectors of infection', transmitting HIV from themselves to their children or from one man (often assumed to be gay or bisexual) to another, with no recognition whatsoever of the fact that the women concerned are themselves ill (for further discussion of this phenomenon, see Paula Treichler's article 'AIDS, Gender and Biomedical Discourse' in Elizabeth Fee and Daniel Fox's book *AIDS – The Burdens of History*). In Thailand, men commonly refer to *any* sexually transmitted disease as a 'woman's disease', and AIDS has become known in that country as a (female) prostitute's disease. There is little evidence to suggest that women who work as prostitutes in the UK are more at risk than other heterosexually active women. Indeed, the opposite is probably nearer the truth, since sex workers tend to be very well informed about sexually transmitted diseases, and to take precautions to prevent becoming infected. In the developed world, prostitute organizations such as COYOTE (Call Off Your Old Tired Ethics) in the USA and the ECP (English Collective of Prostitutes) have organized to educate women working in the sex industry about the practicalities of safer sex, and rates of infection recorded among prostitute women in these countries are in fact very low. In the third world, the safety of women who work in prostitution depends very much on factors outside their control, such as the particular form prostitution takes in their country and the willingness of their government to acknowledge their existence. In countries such as Thailand, where affluent white male 'sex tourists' visit from many European countries (including Britain) for the express purpose of getting as much sex as they can, and where the government, overriding fierce opposition from local women's organizations, has colluded with this, women are very much at risk, and many become infected. In Senegal, an imaginative scheme is working with local prostitute women to set up co-operative sewing and laundry businesses as alternatives to prostitution; in Nigeria, women who work as prostitutes have been recruited as safer sex educators, and the local 'Stop AIDS' scheme has set up health officers in kiosks at stop-off points on the major lorry routes. In India, on the other hand, women working as prostitutes who have tested positive for HIV have been forcibly detained in prison or remand centres, *without* at any time being educated about HIV, their own health or safer sex.

Prostitution is not primarily a moral or legal issue. It is an economic and political one. As long as 'sex' is seen as something which women *are* and men *do*, and as long as women are kept in economic subservience, female prostitution, with all its attendant risks to women's health and men's, will remain inevitable.

Perhaps the nastiest side of female prostitute-blaming is that concern is seldom, if ever, directed towards the women themselves. Rather, attention is focused on the 'threat' they pose to their clients, and by implication, to the 'normal' families and 'decent' wives of those men. The notion that the prostitute woman, rather than the men who pay for her services, represents a risk to the family, a potential source of contamination, is an ancient one. A truly startling feat of irrationality shifts attention and censure from the central figure in the drama, the man who uses both wife and prostitute, to one of his victims. With HIV/AIDS as with syphilis in earlier times, prostitute women, who are, of course, *at* risk from their male clients (many of whom refuse to use condoms or offer more money for intercourse without a condom), are seen only as *being* a risk to 'innocent' men.

It is as though infection may only be said to have occurred once a man has been infected; infecting a woman somehow does not count until she passes it on.

This cruel logic is also deployed against injecting drug users who have passed the virus on to their children. It is apparent too in the decision to screen women attending antenatal clinics in an attempt to ascertain the spread of the epidemic among the general population. Of course all screening carried out for epidemiological purposes (screening refers to mass testing carried out anonymously, to assess the extent of an epidemic rather than in order to diagnose individuals tested) can be said to be ignoring the needs of the individuals tested in favour of the wider needs of the 'general public' for infection control. But the screening of pregnant women takes place against a background of great anxiety about the possibility of women 'infecting' their unborn children, and of an ugly tendency to declare women guilty of infecting 'innocent' children. In this context, the idea of simply using this convenient research population for data collection has a certain vicious irony.

Direct and indirect implications for women's health

HIV/AIDS issues have, for women as for gay men, been mapped on to an already existing picture of social inequalities. For women, as we have seen, this means their having to take on an additional burden of caring, whether as paid workers, as volunteers or within the family. Their particular relationship to the medical industry also means that their own health needs in relation to HIV are seen as secondary to their supposed role as 'transmitters' of infection. There are, too, important ways in which the social position of women makes it more difficult for them to survive the epidemic.

Firstly, the spurious link between homosexuality and AIDS, and the developing familiarity of the articulate middle-class gay man as the archetypal spokesperson-with-AIDS, locks into the existing tendency to perceive men's health problems as 'real' and to pay more attention to men's illnesses. The result is that HIV infection is associated in the minds of many doctors with gay men in particular and social deviants in general. It is simply not easy to believe that the happily married 50-year-old mother of three sitting in your surgery might have HIV. This means that many women infected with HIV are unable to get a correct diagnosis until they are seriously ill, and indeed that many have probably died without their condition ever having been recognized for what it was. Additionally, there is evidence that family doctors concerned to spare their patients the stigma of an AIDS-related diagnosis avoid mentioning HIV or AIDS on death certificates, referring only to the opportunistic infection (such as pneumonia or cancer) which was specifically responsible for death.

This has serious implications for individual women and for health promotion more widely. Clearly, if a woman is infected with HIV, the sooner she is able to have that diagnosed, the sooner she will have access to medical treatments which may alleviate symptoms, cure infections and prolong her life. It is a chilling fact that women die twice as fast as men once diagnosed with AIDS. It has been suggested that this is due to a combination of things that include misdiagnosis based on outmoded ideas of 'risk groups', the tendency (on the part of doctors, friends, family members and the woman herself) not to take women's symptoms seriously, and the practical difficulties women commonly face in making time to get to the doctor. The implications for health promotion are clear. If numbers of women are becoming ill and dying with their HIV status unrecognized or unrecorded, this lends support to those who still argue that AIDS is not worth worrying about unless you are gay or a drug user, and reinforces the (surprisingly widespread) notion that women are not at risk themselves, and that heterosexual men do not need to take action to protect themselves or their partners. Health promotion messages aimed at heterosexuals are thus more likely to be brushed aside or interpreted as alarmist. Additionally, identifying HIV/AIDS as a male medical problem fits into the existing tendency to devote more time and effort to researching men's health issues. Important medical research on HIV, AIDS and women is unfunded or underfunded and just does not get done.

HIV infection seems to have specific medical consequences for women, with a different pattern of opportunistic infections, different survival rates and different transmission risks (women become infected far more readily than men during unprotected penile penetration). There are also specific questions which need to be asked, such as the potential transmission risk represented by menstrual bleeding (for both the woman and her sexual partner), whether the cyclical changes in the physiology of the vagina have implications for safer sex, or whether women's health is put at risk by long term exposure to the side effects of the spermicidal lubricants recommended as prophylaxis against HIV. Most of these lubricants contain Nonoxynol-9, which has been shown in experiments to cause changes in the vaginal cells of rats, and many women report allergic reactions. These concerns seem to be regarded by the medical establishment as a fairly low priority on the research agenda, despite the probability that the inflammation associated with an allergic reaction may make a woman more vulnerable to HIV.

Promoting safer sex

Health promotion will remain, for the foreseeable future, the only means of slowing the epidemic. In this context, the medical profession's reluctance to accept as 'sex' anything which departs from the 'normal' model of penis-in-vagina intercourse makes it very difficult for non-penetrative sex to gain 'official' recognition as the single most effective physical strategy to prevent the transmission of HIV, something which has great importance bearing in mind the degree of esteem and respect in which doctors and the advice they give are held.

However, it is not just, or even mainly, in relation to the medical profession that specific problems arise for women in the context of safer sex, but in the wider social context of women's lives. Women as a group have little economic, social or sexual autonomy relative to men, a situation which is crucial when considering their ability to protect themselves from infection. For example, because women's autonomous sexuality is not recognized or accepted, heterosexual women are assumed to want penetrative sex and lesbian women's need for specific information and/or health care is not understood or met. Even now, many years into the epidemic, there is very little information available which is aimed at women whose sexual partners are women, and much of what is available is based on assumptions about what lesbians need to know. Thus we have the strange and alarming situation where information about potential HIV precautions during cunnilingus are found *only* in material targeted at lesbians, as though this was a practice entirely foreign to heterosexual couples. Dental dams, latex sheets commonly recommended as a barrier to possible infection during cunnilingus, are widely advertised in the lesbian press, while the average heterosexual couple could be forgiven for never having heard of them.

Within heterosexual relationships, it is clear that women are expected to take responsibility for sexual safety generally. Increasingly, contraception has come to be seen as women's business, with women bearing many costs to their health, ranging from constant depression to a perforated uterus, some of which are life-threatening. Meanwhile, as we are reminded by Myriam Miedzian in her book *Boys Will Be Boys* or by Shere Hite's well-known research, their male partners generally feel they have a right to expect trouble-free, spontaneous sex, and are increasingly unlikely to stay around to offer support if contraception goes wrong and pregnancy ensues. Yet again it is then the woman who has to make the decision whether or not to continue with the pregnancy, to persuade doctors either to allow an abortion or to allow her to remain pregnant, to cope with the trauma of termination or the trauma of pregnancy and labour, and, if she goes ahead with the birth, to devote eighteen years of her life to parenting the child or to negotiate the emotional minefield of adoption. The promotion of 'safer sex' as a response to HIV/AIDS has seemed to many women a bitter irony. Sex has never been safe for women. Besides diseases such as herpes, chlamydia, gonorrhoea, syphilis etc., which of course affect men too, women are at risk from rape and sexual violence as well as from the possibility of unwanted pregnancy and abortion, and the sometimes dangerous complications that can be induced by contraception. In the era of a new respectability for the condom, it is not lost on feminist commentators that the same practices which protect against HIV also protect against cervical cancer, something which was known for some years before the start of the HIV/AIDS epidemic. In 1989, 4,496 women in Britain were known to have cervical cancer, of whom 2,170 died (figures from Women's National Cancer Control Campaign). In the same year, another 848 people in Britain developed AIDS, of whom 301 died (figures from CDSC Monthly Report 1990). There is no 'buddying' service for these women, no support systems and counselling, and there has never been a national campaign to promote the kind of safer sex which could have saved their lives.

In fact, the majority of women have very little control over what happens in their heterosexual relationships and encounters. If this were not so, an unwanted pregnancy would be a rare event, not the commonplace happening which it is today. Research such as that carried out by the Women, Risk and AIDS Project at Goldsmith's College of the University of London by Nicola Gavey, a psychologist at the University of Auckland, or by the Society for Women and AIDS in Africa, has shown that heterosexual sex, for the vast majority of the world's women, is more often than not uncomfortable, painful, embarrassing or humiliating, far from pleasurable, and that they are seldom willing and equal partners. Even for the educated and well-informed middle-class woman in the industrialized West, a woman whose peer culture allows her to be assertive and to consider herself the equal of her male partner, the business of negotiating safer sex is recognized to be far from straightforward. Such women (and men) are in a minority even within their own societies. Given that two-thirds of the world's illiterates are women, that women in *all* countries are poorer than men (and thus likely to be economically dependent on them) and that young women are still sold into prostitution by their families in some countries (see Joni Seager and Ann Olson's book *Women in the World*), the idea of equality within heterosexual relationships is simply not a reality for most women.

If women risk a lot by taking part in heterosexual activity, they risk much by refusal. Women may be socially ostracized, turned out by their partner or husband, beaten up, raped or even killed for trying to refuse sex. They may risk losing a relationship on which they are socially and economically as well as emotionally dependent. Sex is widely understood to be something which men do to women, and a service which men feel they have a right to demand of women. This is a picture which is as true of Oxbridge undergraduates as it is of Muslims in Pakistan, of Catholic council tenants in deprived parts of Glasgow or of young Latinos in the USA. It is a picture which is changing, but it is changing for a tiny proportion of couples. 'Negotiation' and 'consent' are concepts which have very little relation to the heterosexual lives of most women. They are concepts which are crucial to the practice of safer sex.

Women are caught in a desperate trap. In the West, most men, linking AIDS with gay sex and anxious to keep their distance from anything contaminated by association with homosexuality, refuse to believe that HIV is a risk for them (as shown, for example, in research carried out by Stephen Clift and his colleagues in Canterbury). Sociological research carried out in response to the HIV epidemic has revealed startling evidence that there are large numbers of men who regularly have sex with other men, while simultaneously clinging to their heterosexual status and self-image. This group of men simply do not link their actions with the lives of the 'poofs' and 'benders' held up to such vociferous derision in the tabloids, and do not pay attention to safer sex messages targeted at the gay community. They are of course unlikely to tell their wives and girlfriends of their sexual encounters with other men.

Surveys, such as that carried out by the National AIDS Trust in 1991, suggest that young women are on the whole more realistic about the risks of HIV than young men (though of course there are women as well as men who dismiss the idea that heterosexuals are at risk). Yet a realistic assessment of risk is not enough unless it is possible to carry out appropriate precautions to reduce that risk. Any woman trying to negotiate safer sex, either by using condoms or by exploring routes to orgasm which do not involve penetration, has the whole ideological weight of 'real' masculinity stacked against her. The gender rules of masculinity are unforgiving and, although under lively challenge from feminists and new men, they are still dominant in Western culture. These informal rules demand full vaginal penetration, orgasm inside a woman (anything else slides threateningly into 'premature ejaculation'), a refusal to comply with anything which interrupts the 'spontaneity' of sexual passion, an anxious identification of sex with 'performance', a belief that a real man should know about sex and that a real woman should be innocent/ignorant and certainly should not tell her man what to do, that a man is powered by a sex drive and may enjoy casual sexual encounters while a woman is more emotional, caring more for 'love' than sex, and is naturally monogamous. It is simply intolerable, within the dictates of this ideology, for a woman to negotiate the use of a condom, let alone non-penetrative sex. At the same time, women (and women's genitals in particular) are culturally associated with contamination and with disease. Women's sexuality is seen as threatening and linked with seduction into powerlessness and death. The ages-old image of sexual woman, as we have seen earlier, is of a deathtrap, as the honey-pot luring men in to die from syphilis, gonorrhoea and now AIDS. So, at the same time as it is made virtually impossible for women to protect themselves and their male sexual partners from the possibility of infection, they are identified as an infection *risk* in themselves, and blamed for 'passing the infection on' to men and babies.

If this seems extreme, it is worth studying the mountain of safer sex promotional materials from both governmental and nongovernmental sources. It is clear that such materials are targeted at specific groups. Nobody would suggest that safer sex material produced for gay men could be used effectively with heterosexual women or vice versa. So this huge pile of material may by and large be categorized according to the target group it is aimed at. Doing this we find that there is plenty for gay men (often produced by gay men themselves), which is by and large glossy, well-produced, sexually explicit and erotic. Sex is depicted as something which is fun, positive and pleasurable, and clear, explicit advice is available to make it safe. Turning to the (fairly sizeable pile) of material aimed at 'women' (usually including lesbian women as an afterthought), we find an immediate difference. For women, sex is depicted as something potentially shocking and embarrassing; indeed, several leaflets on safer sex for women carry prudery warnings on the front, warning you not to read them if you are easily shocked. Either the 'easily shocked' may be left to die, or there is more concern about offending women than about saving their lives! This feeds into the general rule that women must be 'innocent' of sexual desire. Unfortunately, it is this very 'innocence' which makes it inevitable that sex is understood to be something done *by* men, *to* women and probably against their will. Such a view of sex is not one which makes it possible for women to negotiate safer sex. Such health promotional materials are, ironically, doing much to make it harder for women to practise safer sex.

There is another, tiny pile of material specifically aimed at lesbians and lots aimed rather diffusely at 'young people' (largely, though not exclusively, assumed to be heterosexual) or 'drug users' (ditto). There is also some good material produced by the Haemophilia Society for haemophiliacs (all of whom appear, on the evidence of this material, to be heterosexual).

There is a glaring omission from these piles of safer sex information. In all my years working in the field, I have come across only *one* leaflet aimed specifically at heterosexual men. There is plenty of advice to heterosexual women on how to persuade their partner to practise safer sex. There is even a book called *How to Persuade Your Lover to Wear a Condom and Why You Should*. Much mention is made of women being 'assertive', with some writers going so far as to recommend assertiveness training for women to enable them to negotiate their sexual needs (!). This is blatant victim-blaming. To ascribe men's refusal to contemplate safer sex as a failure on the part of women to be assertive is to ignore the social reality of centuries. It is also to continue the tradition of demanding that women take responsibility not only for their own health but for that of their partner, and specifically for the success and safety of heterosexual sex.

The risk for women

Risk from heterosexual sex

Perhaps the most bitter irony of all lies in the fact that, despite being viewed as a 'vector of transmission' of the virus, or a 'risk' to men, or even a 'reservoir of infection', women are more at risk of contracting HIV infection from heterosexual intercourse than their male partners. In the Panos Institute's dossier *Triple Jeopardy*, the writers note that, in the industrialized West, the risk for women may be as much as three times greater than for men (this pattern is also present in some African countries, though is not generally true of the African continent, where equal numbers of women and men appear to be infected). The reason for this is probably straightforwardly mechanical. The semen of an HIV+ man contains a highly infectious quantity of virus, which, whether deposited into the vagina or the rectum, poses a high risk of transmission. Vaginal secretions have also been found to contain infectious quantities of virus, but their route into the male body is less direct (through the opening of the urethra in the glans of the penis, or through minute abrasions on the glans or under the foreskin) and a smaller quantity is generally produced. It has also been suggested that women are more likely to have older, more sexually experienced (the implication is 'and therefore more likely to be infected') partners.

We simply do not know how many people, men and women, have become infected through heterosexual vaginal sex in Britain. The unhelpful practice of cataloguing infected individuals according to their membership of 'risk groups' probably does much to obscure the frequency of heterosexual transmission. The majority of those who inject illegal drugs are heterosexual, and in most cases there is no means of conclusively establishing whether they became infected through sharing contaminated injecting equipment or through unsafe sex. Yet they go on record under the risk category of 'injecting drug user'. Despite widespread popular myths about the stereotypical 'junkie', it is quite probably easier (given the ready availability of new, sterile equipment) for women who inject drugs to practise safer drug use than it is for them to insist on the practice of safer sex in their heterosexual partnerships. And as long as drug users are defined as only or primarily at risk through their injection practices rather than their sexual practices, it will not get any easier for women who inject drugs to protect themselves from contracting HIV sexually.

Increased risk for lesbian women

For lesbian women, HIV/AIDS has had a contradictory and complex history. Many lesbians have been deeply involved from the earliest stages of the epidemic in the gay community response. Lesbians have worked hard on the volunteer help lines, the safer sex information campaigns, the buddying services, the activist and lobbying groups, the fund-raising events, the hospices and welfare advice centres, the training programmes. Lesbian writers, photographers, film-makers, journalists, graphic artists and cartoonists have poured energy into cultural activism, and into the crucial arena of social and cultural commentary which has served to expose the unjust and oppressive practices of many statutory organizations in their response to AIDS.

Yet other lesbians have angrily refused to get involved in HIV/AIDS work, pointing out that the rush to support 'our gay brothers' has all been one way. Where were gay men, they ask, in the battle for abortion rights, the fight against sterilization abuse, the struggle for women's mental health rights, action on the rights of lesbian mothers to have custody of their own children or to control their fertility? What stand have gay men taken on the issues which have long made life dangerous for lesbians and all women, on rape, violence against women, pornography? And after all, they argue, AIDS is not an issue for lesbians.

There is certainly a lot of truth in the complaint that gay men have been noticeably lacking in solidarity and support for health and social policy issues affecting lesbians – the support in the 'lesbian and gay community' has undoubtedly been almost exclusively one-way. In fact, lesbians who are also feminists have good reason to be angry with the disdain, and often public ridicule, heaped on feminism and feminists by certain gay male activists and writers. Yet to assert that AIDS is not an issue for lesbians is dangerously untrue. There may well be conflict in the community between lesbian interests and gay men's interests, but the world outside the community does not stop to consider whether 'homosexual' means male or female. Those who proclaim that AIDS is the just deserts of perversion, or divine retribution on unnatural sex, do not distinguish between male and female 'deviancy'. The increase in anti-gay feeling and activity associated with HIV/AIDS results in increased danger for lesbians as well as for gay men. Overtly AIDS-related attacks have been recorded on lesbians, and the general increase in social intolerance of same-sex relationships in Britain has accorded popular support to directly anti-lesbian legislation.

The fact that lesbians are the group at lowest risk of sexual transmission of HIV has proved a double-edged sword. It is a simple fact that the sexual transmission of HIV from one woman to another is very rare; though the evidence in some recorded cases suggests that it is not entirely impossible. This is of course very different from saying that lesbians 'do not get AIDS'. They do. Lesbians, although defined by heterosexuals on the basis of a sexual preference for other women, are a wide-ranging social group. Lesbians who inject drugs, receive blood transfusions or are exposed to needlestick injuries are not protected from HIV infection by the fact that their sexual partners are female. Additionally, many women become lesbian after years of heterosexual life. Many have been married, some have worked as prostitutes, some continue to work as prostitutes, or simply to have occasional sex with men, even after identifying as lesbian. Clearly, heterosexual intercourse still poses a potential risk for these women, and some may have been infected by previous male partners long before they embarked upon sexual relationships with women.

Sadly, it has sometimes been difficult for lesbians with HIV or AIDS to find the support they need from other lesbians. Since lesbian sex is so safe, women who are infected may be blamed for somehow 'doing something wrong'. It seems that, even within a different ethical and social context, illness may still be associated with wrongdoing and blame.

What has conspicuously *not* happened is a general rush of other groups to the lesbian community to find out just why lesbian sex is so safe, and to ask what others may learn from the lesbian example. Clearly such an idea is unimaginable given the opprobrium and loathing with which 'deviant' sex is regarded within the wider community, and given the social and political threat to the status quo posed by a group of women who are evidently *safer* than 'normal' heterosexual women *because* they do not have sex with men. Yet it is worth recognizing that, were it not for social and political considerations, medical common sense should suggest that any group whose behaviour puts it at risk of contracting a potentially lethal condition could do no better than to seek advice from a group whose behaviour clearly protects it from that condition.

Reproduction and reproductive rights

Because of the way our society is divided along gender lines, paediatric AIDS is seen in the public mind as a women's problem; or, more accurately, women are seen as the problem in paediatric AIDS. The medical facts are not yet clear. It is known that children born to a woman who has HIV or AIDS are at risk of being HIV+ themselves. Research is going on to assess the risks of transmission during pregnancy, during delivery (perhaps by contact with maternal blood) or via breast milk. In the early days of the epidemic, when women were only diagnosed once they were actually ill, and when many women passed through the antenatal clinics and delivery suites with their HIV+ status remaining unsuspected, the picture for

HIV+ women who wished to have children seemed grim. It was thought that the chance of passing on the virus to the baby was very high indeed, that pregnancy exacerbated existing illness and hastened the progression to extreme immune incapacity, and that breast milk was highly infectious. Now, with the benefit of much improved data and with advances in the clinical care of people with HIV, the picture is much less alarming. All babies born to HIV+ women have antibodies to HIV in their blood. This is because the mother's antibodies are present within the baby's blood for some months after birth, during which time the child's own antibodies gradually take over, and the blood chemistry changes. Such babies are given blood tests at regular intervals, to determine whether or not they themselves are infected, and results are much more encouraging than was at first thought. Estimates now suggest that as few as 10–15 per cent of babies born to HIV+ women are themselves infected with the virus.

Similarly, it is now known that pregnancy has little effect on the progression of the mother's HIV illness, though research continues. Regarding breast milk, the World Health Organization quite categorically states that the risks to the baby of bottle-feeding are far greater than the possible risk of HIV transmission via breastfeeding (see *The Third Epidemic*). This is especially true in many developing countries, where the active promotion of artificial feeding by baby-feed companies is responsible for thousands of infant deaths annually, but it is also true in the industrialized West. Although there is a theoretical risk of transmission through breast milk, it is now generally thought to be small. However, a newly delivered mother who has HIV will quite naturally feel a very high degree of concern about the health risks to her child, and may also have to cope with feelings of guilt about the effects on the child of her own possible early illness and/or death. In these circumstances, it takes an act of tremendous faith to breastfeed, however tiny the risk may be. Those responsible for the care and counselling of women in this situation need to be extraordinarily sensitive and well informed.

In the area of reproductive rights, as with any other area touched by HIV/AIDS, the virus does not cause new problems, it merely adds another dimension to problems which already exist. The question of who controls a woman's body has been the site of bitter struggle throughout history, a struggle which is merely intensified by the advent of HIV. The biological baseline is that women can gestate, give birth to and nourish new people, while men cannot. On to this bodily reality, all cultures have attempted to map their own sets of meanings, and out of it all cultures have felt obliged to develop their own social controls and institutions. The key issue they shared seems to have been how to establish some power and control over this vital process *for men*, and the point we have reached in late twentieth-century Britain is that women have, in point of fact, very little autonomous control over their bodies, their sexuality or their reproductive potential (as the public struggles over abortion, 'virgin' birth, the provision of donor insemination to lesbians and the stigmatizing of 'pretended families' explicit in Section 28 of the 1988 Local Government Act demonstrate).

There is not space here to delineate the fascinating and at times horrific history of this struggle as it has been enacted in different eras, in different countries and within the paradigms of different religions, beliefs and cultures. What is crucial is that we recognize that, when she contemplates any course of action within the area of sexuality or reproduction, a woman is obliged to set her own feelings, wishes and needs against a wide range of social structures and institutions which prioritize the wishes of men. Thus, if she does not have a partner and wishes to become pregnant, society will regard that wish as unnatural, immoral, deviant or even criminal, and she will have a real fight on her hands if she wants medically competent help to fulfil it. To become pregnant via 'informal' methods always carried an alarming risk since, if a man can prove he was the biological father of a woman's child, he is accorded important rights by law, and could theoretically demand custody, even of a child he had had no contact with for many years. If the woman concerned is a lesbian, the prospect of being judged an 'unfit mother' by the courts is a very real one, and the fear of losing a deeply loved child to its biological father is therefore great. Many lesbian women have, therefore, approached gay men for this purpose, since they were thought less likely to demand in the future that their paternity rights be recognized. With the advent of HIV, this becomes much more problematic, and women are increasingly obliged to approach formal bodies such as the Pregnancy Advisory Service (PAS) if they wish to become pregnant using donated sperm. (In 1991 PAS announced that it was no longer making its services available to lesbian women. It denies that government pressure was in any way involved in this decision.)

Similarly, the issue of abortion is largely about men's control over women's bodies, and as such, is deeply entwined with issues such as class, race and dis/ability. While articulate middle-class women often have to fight to be allowed a termination, women whom the medical profession rejects as 'unfit to breed', such as women of colour, poor working-class women and women with physical and/or cognitive disabilities, often have to fight to be allowed to continue a pregnancy which the *doctor* (usually male) deems to be a problem. On the other hand, as groups such as Women's Health (formerly Women's Health and Reproductive Rights Campaign) have discovered, such women may find, when they do need a termination, that they are offered one only on the condition that they agree to be sterilized.

The history of scientific medicine and fertility control is shadowed by the eugenicist movement of the first half of this century. The clearest examples of eugenicist abuse come from the USA. Angela Y. Davis, in her book *Women, Race and Class*, tells how, as recently as the 1970s, thousands of Black, Latina and Native American women were coercively sterilized by US governmental programmes, as were women labelled as mentally 'deficient' or mentally ill, often before they had had any children at all. Frequently these women were simply not told what was being done to them, while in other cases, the welfare benefits which kept families from starving were only paid to the family if the daughters were sterilized. Many young women were told that the process was a temporary one, a lie which naturally caused enormous distress and misery as they were eventually obliged to realize that they would never be able to have children.

On to this bitter and painful history, HIV/AIDS has fallen like a lead weight. Women who have HIV are subject to multiple stigma in the eyes of the medical profession. To the stigma of being female, with all its associations with contamination and pathology, is added that of simply having HIV, with yet further stigma if you are or have been an injecting drug user or if you have contracted the virus during sex with someone you were not married to. This is, I must stress, *not* to say that all doctors behave like little Hitlers. There are many thoroughly open-minded, thoroughly professional, thoroughly good and supportive doctors and other health care workers caring for women with HIV infection, and their compassion and sensitivity are unquestionable. I have come into contact with many such men and women, and would sing their praises unstintingly. But health care professionals come in all shapes and sizes, and it is sadly true that *in general* women with HIV come up against the same problems with their medical carers as all women. Women with HIV have been urged not to become pregnant, have been pressured into terminating wanted pregnancies, have been regarded as irresponsible if they became pregnant knowing their HIV status, and have been warned not to breastfeed.

For the woman drug user, condemnation is widespread. Women who inject drugs have long been blamed for the drug-related health problems of their babies, an attitude which shows real ignorance about drug addiction. After all, how many mothers-to-be who smoke find it easy to give up during pregnancy? If you add to the physiological nature of chemical dependency the complex social issues which surround doing something which is illegal, which is embedded in a specific sub-culture, and which may have particular effects on your health, your emotions, your personality and your way of life, the idea that drug users have a choice ('just say no') is clearly simplistic and insultingly judgemental. If it is that simple, if 'saying no' is that powerful, then why does the Health Education Authority have to spend such huge sums in the fight to get us to give up cigarettes?

Given the atrocity-ridden history of women's fight for bodily autonomy, and for reproductive rights in particular, some feminists are predicting worst-case scenarios in relation to AIDS which are truly alarming. How long will it be, they wonder, before women are forcibly tested before they become pregnant, with those testing positive being sterilized and those testing negative urged to have more children than they perhaps want, to replenish the stock of 'uncontaminated' individuals? How long before a negative HIV test becomes a 'dowry', something which defines only uninfected women as marriageable? If this seems utterly beyond the realms of possibility, it is chilling to remember that prostitute women in Thailand are currently issued with certificates showing the result of an HIV antibody test, and the punters are officially warned not to have sex with women who cannot produce evidence of a negative test. The contact ads in the US gay press, full of euphemisms like 'healthy' and in some cases actually proclaiming 'antibody negative', already bear witness to the suggestion that for some people, evidence of HIV status influences their choice of sexual partner or potential mate.

Not simply a 'women's problem'

It is abundantly clear that, for women around the world as in the UK, the medical problem of HIV/AIDS has to be seen as another problem they have about men. In the context of this epidemic, men represent an intransigent risk for women. As long as men continue to rape it will not be possible for any woman, whether 1 year old or 91 years old, to reassure herself that she is not at risk from HIV. As long as men feel justified in making such a fuss about condoms, as long as they continue offering women more to have sex without a condom (whether 'more' means more money, more love, more commitment), the risk to women is outside their control. As long as women remain economically and socially subordinate to men, women will have little negotiating power within heterosexual relationships. As long as a multi-billion-pound pornography industry continues to promote penetration and to represent women as creatures who have sex done to them by men, women will find it impossible to get their sexual needs, including safer sex, taken seriously. As long as men, whether gay or straight, insist on their innate need for the 'release of sexual tension' and their right to have casual sex on their terms, men's beliefs about male sexual need will simply conflict with women's needs for sexual safety (and, ironically, with men's safety too where HIV is concerned). As long as the streets and public spaces of our towns and cities are seen as sexual playgrounds by some men (whether they be heterosexual men sexually intimidating passing women or kerb crawling in red light districts, or gay men meeting or having sex in cruising areas), women will be seen as legitimate prey if they venture into that 'playground', and their sexual autonomy will not exist.

If safer sex is to be widely adopted, and remember, that is the *only* strategy we have against this dreadful epidemic, then such social issues must be tackled. If they are not, there is little chance of slowing the steady increase in infection rates among heterosexuals, men as well as women. So far, by targeting women and gay men with safer sex messages and by totally ignoring the difficult issue of how to target heterosexual men, health promotion initiatives, whether statutory or voluntary, have simply added to the problem. We will all pay for that cowardice.

4

Green monkeys and dark continents: AIDS and racism

Although there is a general recognition among more thoughtful people that categorizing AIDS as the 'gay plague' is both wrong and offensive, there is still a widely held belief in something equally suspect called 'African AIDS'. Many who consider themselves well informed still subscribe to the (discredited) belief that HIV/AIDS came from Africa. This outmoded belief is often accompanied by a whole set of wildly inaccurate generalizations about the 'epidemic in Africa'. Left-wing gay activist Peter Tatchell, for example, is not immune from statistical 'creativity', asserting that 'In Africa it is estimated that 6 per cent of the total population is now infected.' In 1986, when Tatchell published this piece of misinformation in *7 Days* (18 October), WHO records report no more than 1,069 cases of AIDS from Africa as a whole. Africa has a population of around 517 million, so if Tatchell's figures are correct, 31 million people in Africa in 1986 would have had HIV. Even the most pessimistic accounts do not suggest more than a hundred undiagnosed HIV infections per one case of AIDS; Tatchell's figure would result in a ratio of HIV infection to recorded AIDS cases of 29,000 to one! Where do such ideas originate, and why are they still so widely held to be true?

One favourite theory (among white commentators) of the origins of HIV/AIDS goes as follows: HIV is a mutation of a similar virus which is found in African green monkeys and was somehow passed on to humans. It was taken to Haiti by migrant Black workers, who infected a 'pool' of Haitian male prostitutes, who then infected US gay men vacationing in Haiti. The US gay men, the story continues, because of their sexual promiscuity and ready access to international travel, sparked off the epidemic in the first world. Although this theory was based on very flimsy evidence, and has since been rejected by some of the scientists who originally suggested it, it achieved instant popularity with the press and media and received widespread publicity. Maps showing the putative global route taken by the epidemic as dramatic arrows radiating from the heart of Africa became commonplace in books, magazines, newspapers and television documentaries. So what truth is there in the theory that HIV originated in Africa? Probably none.

As Haringey Council's Race Equality Unit records, in its paper *AIDS and Racism*, sophisticated genetic tests have now indicated that the virus which infects green monkeys is fundamentally different to HIV, so different as to discredit claims that one is a mutation of the other. Epidemiological studies, meanwhile, have led researchers to conclude that there is no evidence to suggest that the virus was present in Africa at an earlier time than in the United States. Dr Richard Tedder, a virologist at the Middlesex Hospital, states, 'I find no evidence of this being an archival virus in Africa. Prevalence rates in the African continent started to go up at about the same time as they did in America and Europe.' HIV, in other words, is as recent an arrival in Africa as it is elsewhere in the world. Indeed, some commentators suggest that there is just as much evidence to suggest that the virus was 'exported' from the USA to Africa in supplies of blood and blood products. Although I am emphatically *not* suggesting that this is the case, it is clearly important to recognize that while one of these competing explanations has been widely publicized (and the African origins story is consequently a familiar one to most people in Britain), the other has not.

There is no consensus among the scientific community about the geographical origins of HIV, and the green monkey hypothesis has been resoundingly disproved, yet although many British newspapers, books and television news broadcasts and documentaries have published detailed accounts of this nasty little fiction, there has been a noticeable lack of public correction or retraction. Only one television documentary, *Monkey Business*, broadcast late at night on Channel 4 in 1989, offered a detailed rejection of the green monkey hypothesis – only to replace it with the suggestion that the CIA were responsible for developing HIV in their germ warfare laboratories. Why is something as tenuous as the association between Africa and AIDS met with such wholesale credulity?

The white man's grave

The positioning of Africa in Western accounts of the epidemic can only be understood in the historical context of colonialism, slavery and social Darwinism. The white nations who invaded the African continent, who set about systematically destroying local culture and the local economy, who set in motion the shameful barbarity of the slave trade and who later imposed the grossly inappropriate values and structures of Victorian capitalism on the people whose world they had done their best to destroy, were obliged to justify their actions to themselves and the folks back home. If Africans were recognized as human beings, with a civilization, religious beliefs and 'high' feelings, the wholesale destruction wreaked upon them would be exposed for the barbarism which it in fact was. So the politically and socially expedient notion of the 'savage', a creature lower down the evolutionary ladder than 'civilized' white people, was deployed, and Africa was labelled the Dark Continent, an embodiment of all that was untamed, wild, uncontrollable, bestial and dangerous. Additionally, the early colonists, ill prepared for the climate and environment of Africa, and unprotected by natural immunity or medical prophylaxis, sickened and died in great numbers from unfamiliar diseases.

For whites growing up in Britain in the first half of the twentieth century, the familiar image of Africa and Africans was an uncompromising legacy from the ideology of colonialism. Africa was represented as a huge, hot, undifferentiated and oppressive chaos, which dedicated and masterful white people were struggling to bring under the yoke of civilization. It was swarming with flies, dirt and horrific diseases, and its people were ignorant savages who worshipped idols, let their babies die and killed the missionaries and doctors who tried to help them. Men like Albert Schweitzer and Dr

Livingstone, together with the swarms of missionaries sent out to bring the pitiful savage under the rule of god, were the heroes of Africa. There was a strong thread of uncontrolled sexuality running through these accounts, reflecting the British dread of sex. Africans did not wear clothes and they did not know that you had to be married in order to have sex; African men had huge penises, and were likely to offer a white man a cow in exchange for a white woman to add to their collection of wives.

It is tempting to see this ridiculous and insulting picture as an outmoded leftover, something as archaic as whalebone stays, and as risible. But such vigorously promoted fictions do not simply relinquish their hold on the mind when exposed to the cold light of reality, as the ready welcome offered to the 'African origins of AIDS' fiction indicates. Such an account, devoid of rigorous scientific proof, is only credible in the context of the archaic and racist fictions of colonialism. It is only comprehensible to the racist imagination. Thus the findings in one of the London hospitals early in 1992, showing that a high percentage of pregnant women testing positive for HIV antibodies during a screening programme had connections with Africa, were given copious press coverage. The voice of reason, cautioning that generalizations could not and should not be drawn from one survey undertaken in one hospital (and pointing out that, after all, an even greater percentage of the women sampled had connections with London and had had heterosexual sex!), had little chance of being heard over the determination to justify the familiar narrative of racism.

Monkeying around

The idea that a virus could be passed from monkeys to Black Africans (nobody had ever suggested that white Africans were involved) implies either a clear biological similarity between Black Africans and monkeys, or some vaguely disgusting kind of contact between them. Indeed, *Africa Report* (November/December 1988) records that the South African media, under apartheid, published claims that AIDS was due to ritual and sexual contact between Black Africans and baboons. Such outlandish suggestions find ready agreement in the racist imagination. Research carried out by Jenny Kitzinger and David Miller in 1991 shows that people from all walks of life believe that Africans have sex with animals, including bulls, gorillas and monkeys. Some of their interviewees went further, blaming 'Pakis' having sex with gorillas or monkeys for 'bringing it [AIDS] here'.

Such statements reveal non-white cultures to be an imaginary world constructed, as it were, from the 'missing bits' of white culture, almost a looking-glass reversal where anything might happen. This is hardly surprising, given that people are obliged to fall back on their imagination to construct for them a workable mental model of anything about which they do not have ready access to alternative sources of information. Television is overwhelmingly the most powerful (and credible) source of information in most people's lives. It is certainly cited by most British people as their major source of information about AIDS. Yet British television offers us a picture of Africa which is both limited and distorted. We are obliged to flesh out the bones of an Africa culturally constructed from Tarzan films, wildlife documentaries, brief film clips from television news items about famine, civil war or disaster, and compassion-a-thons such as Live Aid and Comic Relief. With precious little information to balance the scenes of famine, drought and nomadic despair, it is perhaps not surprising that otherwise intelligent people in Britain find it hard to believe the truth that not all Africans live in mud huts in jungles positively teeming with monkeys, that actually the majority seldom see a monkey.

In fact, the pattern of the epidemic in Africa is not quite as different from that in Europe and the USA as we would like to believe. It is not true, for example, that HIV is most prevalent in rural areas (where monkeys are common); rather, HIV infection and AIDS are most often found in towns and cities, as is the case in the UK. Yet, to judge by media representations in the UK, there *is* no urban Africa. It is perhaps salutary to recognize that many Africans are much more aware of the realities of the relationship between Africa and the (over)developed nations than most people in Europe. In some African countries, the local dialect word for AIDS is the same as that for foreign aid.

How bad is the epidemic in Africa?

The same racist imagination paints a lurid and inaccurate picture of the epidemic in Africa, to such a degree that many people believe that 'AIDS is rife' throughout the continent, that whole populations are dying, and that widespread sexual promiscuity combined with peculiar sexual practices is to blame. In fact, of course, Africa is not one country, with one epidemic. Rather, it is made up of many nations with many differing rates and patterns of spread, exactly like Europe. How many British people would be happy for Romania to be taken as the best example of what happens in Europe? Different nations in the African continent may have barely comparable standards of living, economic structures, languages, health care systems or social mores, and it is simply not true that they share one epidemic. Reported cases of AIDS across the 53 African countries vary from 0.3 per million in Nigeria to 568 per million in Congo, with a handful of countries where no cases have been reported at all. The average rate of AIDS cases taken over Africa as a whole is around 78.1 per million, compared to an average taken across the United States of 464 per million, a figure which equals that of Uganda. There are only four countries in Africa which have reported numbers of AIDS cases as bad as, or worse than, the USA. In comparison, the United Kingdom reports 48 cases of AIDS per million, Ireland 31, France 145 and Spain 158. The WHO estimates that half of the global total of 283,010 cases of AIDS are in the United States, a quarter in sub-Saharan Africa and 14 per cent in Europe (figures taken from reports to the World Health Organization by 1 September 1990).

There are reasons to be cautious about such figures, of course. Crucially, they represent the number of cases of AIDS in a country, not the numbers of people with HIV. It is not possible to state categorically how many cases of HIV infection we may expect for every diagnosed case of AIDS, and estimates vary widely. However, it is probably a cautious estimate to suggest that there may be ten people with HIV for every one person diagnosed with AIDS. On the basis of the best figures available, the WHO estimates (1991) that there are a million HIV+ people in North America, a further million in Latin America, close to half a million in Africa and five hundred thousand in Europe. This implies that the situation in Uganda (or the USA), with a likely rate of infection of 4,640 per million, is certainly very grave. Additionally, the number of cases reported is almost certainly an underestimate in most countries, for a variety of reasons. In a wealthy country like Britain, AIDS may go undiagnosed because the patient does not fall into one of the misleading 'risk groups', or may go unreported in an attempt to avoid social stigma. In a very poor country, where the annual health care budget per head of population may be as low as £4–£5, diagnostic technology may not be widely available, many people may simply live too far away from medical centres to get help, local healing traditions may take precedence over Western medicine, or an individual may not be able to take time off from the essentials of subsistence living to seek medical attention. Additionally, people already living at the limit of their physical strength, their health taxed by overwork, malnutrition and frequent exposure to infections and parasites, are likely to become ill and to die very rapidly, before there is time to start the often complex practicalities of consulting a doctor.

On the other hand, some experts have claimed that the situation in many African countries may have been exaggerated. Malaria, for example, frequently gives a false positive result on an HIV antibody test, as do certain other infections and conditions. Testing to eliminate all such possibilities is not feasible when operating under the constraints of poorly resourced and understaffed health services.

Whether the figures are accurate or not, it is clear that the progress of the epidemic is not comparable across all African countries, any more than across all European countries. Nevertheless, it is obvious that someone who becomes infected with HIV in a poor country in central Africa, or in one of the areas where civil wars are being fought, has a very different outlook from someone in a wealthy family in central London. The numbers may not be as high as they are in the United States, but the implications of AIDS for some African nations are nevertheless devastating.

The health consequences of colonialism

This is not the place to detail the complex outline of the impact of colonialism on African countries. Other writers have identified the many negative consequences which colonial exploitation has had for the health of Black Africans. Far from being the Black people's saviour from disease, the white invaders in fact disrupted complex strategies developed over centuries by indigenous peoples to prevent diseases such as sleeping sickness from taking hold. They also introduced new and previously unknown diseases (such as syphilis), and the migrant labour schemes they imposed brought malnutrition and general immiseration to the populations they controlled. The contemporary picture is no better. Black workers in white-owned mines have high rates of respiratory infections, or are vulnerable to the toxic effects of substances such as uranium, while entire nations which have been coerced into replacing agricultural self-sufficiency with cash-crop farming (producing luxury goods such as coffee for the European market) find their economies disastrously tied to the vagaries of world markets and multinational corporations, while their agricultural production is obliged to wrestle with all the problems associated with monoculture, such as pest control and soil exhaustion.

It is against this background that the impact of AIDS on Africa must be seen. If you are lucky enough to live in one of the wealthier African countries, whose cities are large and cosmopolitan, and if you are lucky enough to have a well-paid job and a good education, you will have access to health care as good as any in the North, and your general health is likely to be as good as, or better than, that of someone in a similar position in Paris, Madrid or London. If you were to contract HIV, sophisticated diagnostic and therapeutic support would be available to you.

If you are unlucky enough to live in a rural subsistence community in one of the poorer countries, the story is very different. In such countries, there are not enough trained doctors to go round, the most basic medical necessities are in short supply, and essentials that are taken for granted in Britain, like clean drinking water, fresh foods or even soap, are hard to come by. Testing equipment needed to diagnose HIV is costly, and must be bought at the expense of other, perhaps more urgently needed equipment. To provide new, sterile syringes and needles for every injection or blood test for every patient (a procedure taken for granted in British clinics and hospitals) would eat up most of the annual health care budget, so injecting equipment must perforce be re-used. The drugs used to postpone deterioration of the immune system in people with HIV, or to combat the various opportunistic infections associated with AIDS, are very costly, and might just as well be on Mars as far as most third world countries are concerned. Uganda, for example, one of the worst affected countries, had in 1988 an annual AIDS budget of less than $5 million. AZT, the drug most widely used in the USA to prolong the life of people with HIV/AIDS, cost in 1988 $10,000 per patient per year. This stark economic equation holds true, of course, for any eventual cure or vaccine which may be developed. In other words, it is not the 'promiscuity' or strange sexual practices of Darkest Africa which have resulted in the rapid spread of HIV in some African countries; it is poverty.

It is important to stress this, because experience has shown that many white British people who should know better hold very bizarre views about the sexual behaviour of Black Africans. A Radio 4 phone-in host was the centre of a small storm in 1991 when he hung up in disgust on a (male) caller who said, vis-à-vis Black Africans and AIDS, 'Well, we just don't know what goes on in those mud huts, do we?' It is tempting to write such blatant nonsense off as the thoughtless prejudice of an ill-educated few, but such views (albeit less crudely expressed) have been aired in surprising places. Thus in *AIDS*, a textbook about HIV/AIDS for younger schoolchildren by Alison and David Kilpatrick, we find the statement that: 'In central Africa, heterosexual men are generally more promiscuous than in Europe and America, and going to a prostitute is more socially acceptable. It seems likely that prostitutes in particular, and promiscuous behaviour generally, have made central Africa the most AIDS-ridden area in the world.' (The same book tells us that the only reason lesbians are a 'low risk group' is that they are seldom promiscuous. This husband-and-wife team clearly has a moral message to promote!)

It is clear that, while such unsubstantiated and offensive rubbish is being taught in our schools, health promotion which aims to equip everyone with the knowledge and motivation to protect themselves from HIV infection is fighting a losing battle. Just as homophobia is proving lethal to heterosexuals in the context of HIV/AIDS, so racism is proving potentially lethal to those whose prejudice and bigotry overrules logic and understanding.

One man's promiscuity

Even in the august pages of the *Guardian* we have become accustomed to read of the promiscuity rife in Africa, and the particular threat posed by African prostitute women. It was the *Guardian* (3 February 1987) which told us of the strange habits of the 'Nairobi hooker' who 'emerges after dark' to 'preen' and to 'stalk her prey'. Once again the magic wand of journalism transforms a vulnerable group of people into nothing less than a predatory monster. There are, too, particular problems in trying to describe Africa from a peculiarly European moral standpoint. It is quite inappropriate to talk about marriage, fidelity, promiscuity, prostitution or sexual identity as if these words described some kind of universal human 'reality'. It should be easy enough to recognize that even within British culture, 'promiscuity' is a word which has shifted meaning dramatically in the last two or three generations, and that 'marriage' means quite different things to different groups of people. The notion of 'prostitution' is a particularly slippery one, since the provision of sexual services for money is one which may be said to include everything from lawful marriage to soliciting on the street. If such wide variations coexist within British culture, how realistic is it to describe African culture in British terms?

In fact, traditional African society is structurally very different from the European model. Greater stress is placed on lineage than on marriage, and the basic social unit is a woman and her children, rather than a heterosexual couple. A man commonly marries a woman very much younger than himself, women abstain from sex after childbirth for a period lasting several months or even years, and the European concept of illegitimacy is not thought significant. This ancient and long-lasting system has proved to be an extremely effective one, although of course it has been stamped out in those parts of the continent which have been subject to Islamic or Christian dominance. There is no justification for asserting that traditional African sexual mores are any more likely to 'spread HIV' than European ones. The key risk factors (as far as it is possible to generalize across a continent) appear to be living or working in an urban environment, having unprotected penetrative sex (both equally true in Europe or the USA) or suffering from genital lesions (STD infection also appears to be an additional risk factor in Europe and the USA). Above all, poverty looms large as a key risk factor for HIV in Africa; the epidemic follows, for example, the path of the great roadways used by long-distance truckdrivers and by the women for whom no survival option other than prostitution is available.

Racism and AIDS in Africa

A very clear indication of the fact that HIV is less of a medical problem than a social and political one comes from South Africa. Here, in a country where racism has long been enshrined in legislation under the policy of apartheid, the impact of institutional racism on health far outweighs other factors. Under apartheid, Blacks and whites are treated in different hospitals and clinics, and are provided with health care under totally different and separate systems. Thus, in 1986, as HIV infection spread throughout the country, the state spent $19 per patient per day in Baragwanath Hospital in the Black township of Soweto, while it spent $88 per day on a similar white patient in the Johannesburg General Hospital. Whites have a doctor–patient ratio of 1:330, while for Blacks the ratio is 1:1,200. In the 'homelands' the situation is bleaker still, with the worst ratio being one doctor per 19,000 patients in Gazankulu (figures from *Africa Report*, November/December 1988). The much vaunted reforms of apartheid have yet to make a significant impact on this grotesque inequality.

The impact of this oppression on health is profound. Blacks have an average life expectancy of 58.9 years, whites 73.2 years. White South Africans live one of the most privileged lifestyles in the world, with an infant mortality rate lower than that of whites in the United States: 14 deaths in the first year of life per thousand births, as compared to 17 in the USA, while the infant mortality rate for Black South Africans is nearer 90 per thousand. The poverty of Black life is reflected in malnutrition, the major cause of infant death, which kills thirty times more Black than white children annually. Diseases of poverty such as tuberculosis, polio and cholera come with the appalling living conditions of the Black communities, and outbreaks of bubonic plague and measles (which kills two million children a year in the developing world) are frequent. In this context, HIV is one more burden which hits the poorest Blacks disproportionately hard, one more load on a health care system already struggling against the odds.

In South Africa, the pattern of HIV infection among the white community appears to follow the pattern familiar from studies of Europe and the USA. The gay male community in the urban areas is among the hardest hit, with heterosexual transmission rates rising at a later date. Among the Black community, the pattern reflects the general picture within the continent, with equal numbers of men and women being infected, and unprotected heterosexual sex the commonest transmission route. There can be no clearer indication of the importance of social issues, including poverty and prejudice, in shaping the epidemic and determining who is 'at risk'.

A disease of poverty

A pattern is emerging in many countries across the globe linking HIV with poverty. And, of course, it is important to remember that poverty is not an African phenomenon, or even exclusive to the third world. In the United States, the richest country in the world, queues at charity-run soup kitchens are steadily lengthening, as poverty on a scale previously only seen in the shanty towns of Brazil follows inexorably on the heels of monetarist economic policy. Part of

Edinburgh was declared a third world development area by the WHO in 1992, while an estimated 36 per cent of the population of Britain are currently living at or below supplementary benefit level, according to the Child Poverty Action Group. Bearing in mind the utter inadequacy of supplementary benefit, it is obvious that many people living marginally above this official poverty line are in fact living in poverty. Hand in hand with poverty come poor nutrition, poor housing, a lowered general standard of health, lower resistance to infection, depression and despair. As long ago as 1980, the Black Report commissioned by the Callaghan Labour government identified clear and incontrovertible links between poverty and ill health, and HIV fits into this familiar picture.

There is, of course, a world of difference between poverty in Britain and poverty in a developing country in central Africa. The very poorest in Britain still have access to a health care service which is (for the time being at any rate) free at the point of delivery. The NHS is not yet in such dire straits that injection equipment must be shared between dozens of patients, and the benefits system, while grossly inadequate, does on the whole prevent people actually dying from starvation. Yet it is as true in Britain as in central Africa (or in the USA for that matter) that poverty hits disproportionately many social groups who are already marginalized. Thus, in Britain and in the USA, the insidious processes of institutionalized racism ensure that people of colour are more likely to be living in poverty than whites. This is reflected in HIV/AIDS statistics, which show that, in the USA, a Latina woman is nine times more likely than a white woman to contract HIV, while a Black woman (African-American) is twelve times more likely.

Racism and AIDS in Britain

Overt racism has touched almost every aspect of the British re-sponse to the epidemic. This is seen most clearly in the enthusiastic acceptance of the African origins story, and in subsequent health promotion efforts. Thus, in 1987, the Terrence Higgins Trust produced an informative booklet, 'AIDS and HIV: Medical

Briefing', which listed, under the heading 'Who can get HIV infection?', 'People having sex with people who have lived in or visited central Africa', commenting that 'anyone who has lived there or visited the area and had sexual intercourse there could ... be at risk'. There was no mention of the potential risks of visiting certain cities in the United States and having sexual intercourse there, despite the fact that, statistically, the likelihood of becoming infected with HIV while visiting some US cities was much greater than in some central African countries! (THT subsequently apologized for this, after a Black woman pointed it out publicly at a conference.) Similarly, the blood transfusion service publicly advises that 'Men and women who have had sex at any time since 1977 with men or women living in African countries, except those on the Mediterranean ... must *not* give blood.' It does not take long for a supposed risk attached to those who have had sex with Africans to be expanded within the racist imagination to include all people with a black skin. Thus, the medical correspondent of *The Times*, Dr Stuttard, publicly labelled young Afro-Caribbean men *living in Britain* as a high risk group in the spread of HIV, an illogical statement based on absolutely no scientific evidence whatsoever, and clearly racist.

The effect on white people of believing that HIV/AIDS is

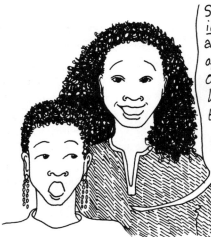

something which is more likely to affect Black people is dangerous in the same way as the belief among some heterosexuals that HIV only affects gays. It is a relief to be able to believe that AIDS is just one more disaster taking place in distant Africa, familiar stage for disease and death. Once the association has been created between blackness and HIV, white people are less likely to see themselves as at risk, and less likely to take steps to protect themselves. Additionally, blackness is seen as intrinsically contaminating within the colonialist logic of racism, in much the same way as homosexuality is seen as intrinsically contaminating within the logic of heterosexism, or female prostitution (and female sexuality generally) as intrinsically contaminating within the logic of sexism. Black people have long been associated in the white racist imagination with animality, perverse and insatiable sexuality and feckless irresponsibility. With a sigh of relief, the chaste white onlooker is now able to imagine HIV as the logical consequence of such behaviour, so different from that of our own dear queen and all her subjects. Once 'risk' has been ascribed to a group so demonstrably alien, a now familiar warped logic demands that those identified as 'at risk' become perceived as posing a risk to others. So, assured on all sides that Black people are at risk for HIV/AIDS, white people are less likely to protect themselves against HIV, or to call for steps to be taken to support and protect the Blacks they believe to be at risk, and more likely to attempt to protect themselves from *the risk to their own health* which they believe Black people to represent.

The implications of the racist response to HIV/AIDS are, therefore, far more dangerous to Black people than to white people. Indeed, reports from many countries indicate that Black people have been subjected to abuse, increased discrimination and even violence related to the belief that they are in some way responsible for AIDS. Thus, African students at Hangzhou University in China were harassed and isolated by their colleagues as a result of the conviction that contact with Black Africans could transmit HIV; Belgian parliamentary spokesman Paul van Stallen proclaimed that 'We shouldn't pay others to come here and be a danger for our own people', as Belgium decided to test African students for HIV; and all African students at one Russian medical school were compulsorily

tested (examples taken from *The Third Epidemic*). In Britain, the
National Front have distributed a leaflet, entitled 'Conspiracy to
Destroy our Nation through AIDS', which asserts that 'AIDS-
infested Africans are brought into Britain from AIDS-infested
Africa ... to live on the dole and social security etc. (at our expense).'
Racism takes its toll on the mental and physical health of all
people of colour living in white society, and HIV once again may be
fitted into a pre-existing picture of oppression and disadvantage.

Racism in health promotion

We are living through a global epidemic whose final toll we may
only guess at, and our only weapon against this epidemic is health
education. Surely, then, it is the basic right of everyone to have
accurate, adequate and sensitive education about HIV and AIDS,
and to have access to the support they may need to enable them to
put health education advice into practice? Yet Black and minority
ethnic groups have been very poorly served by health education in
the UK, despite the fact that their taxes too pay for the health
promotion campaigns which consistently ignore their needs.

Black and minority ethnic workers are underrepresented in both
statutory and voluntary AIDS organizations, and are not adequately
consulted or involved in the planning of major health education
initiatives or the provision of services. There is a lack of educational
material available in languages other than English, and little material or training available on different cultures or religions to guide
HIV/AIDS trainers and educators. Clearly, when working with that
most sensitive of all issues, sex and sexuality, consideration of
cultural and religious beliefs is vital. The safer sex advice which will
be appropriate to a Catholic will be very different from what would
be appropriate to a Protestant, a Muslim, a Jew, an atheist, a
Methodist, a Hindu, a Sikh or a Bahai. Yet there has been no
proliferation of safer sex information carefully tailored to meet the
needs of different religious groups in the UK. It is all too easy to
allow stereotypical ideas about the religious beliefs of different
cultures to become an excuse for not attempting to reach certain

communities with information about safer sex. 'I'm not the right person to do this, I'm not a Hindu/Sikh/Jew' becomes a superficially liberal way of refusing to consider the needs of minority religious or cultural groups.

The interaction of prejudices

The situation of lesbians and gay men of colour is substantially different from that of white lesbians and gay men. In order to survive and resist the damaging effects of racism, strength must be drawn from both family and community. Yet there is no less anti-gay prejudice and bigotry within Afro-Caribbean or Asian families than in the white community. It is not uncommon for homosexuality to be thought of as an exclusively white phenomenon, much as it was labelled the product of Western capitalist decadence in cold war communist regimes. Additionally, in cultures where the family is of central importance, an importance highlighted by the need to maintain integrity and cultural autonomy in the face of white racism, the news that a family member is lesbian or gay brings the recognition that they are probably unlikely to produce children. There is one strand of radical Black political thought which identifies homosexuality as a white perversion which is genocidal to Black families. (It is important to recognize that many white lesbians and gay men report that their parents respond to their revelation of their sexuality by expressing disappointment, grief and anger at being denied grandchildren, a response which often includes the fear that the family name will die out.) There is very little support available for lesbians and gay men of any skin colour, but the consequences of being rejected by one's family are likely to be particularly painful and damaging for lesbians and gays of colour. For a Black or Asian gay man in the UK with HIV/AIDS, the support and care of his family may be particularly important as he struggles with the triple stigma of colour, sexuality and HIV.

For all lesbians and gay men of colour, there is the double burden of racism and homophobia. The visible gay community is largely white, and not especially remarkable for any success in eradicating racism. Black workers who have produced safer sex materials aimed at Black gay men report resistance to their attempts to distribute such materials in both Black and gay community venues. Additionally, although there have been initiatives aimed at providing information about HIV and AIDS in languages such as Bengali, Gujerati or Cantonese, material aimed at lesbians or gay men is not widely available in these languages. It is as though it is only possible to consider one 'ism' at a time. You may be gay, *or* you may be 'ethnic'; you cannot be both at once.

Conclusion

Racism, along with all the other 'isms', acts to speed the progress of the epidemic, not to halt it. It impedes the process of recognizing that all are at risk, thereby putting dangerous obstacles in the way of health education. The legacy of racist colonialist exploitation acts to hasten the progress of the virus across the poor countries in central Africa, while ensuring that the valuable lessons to be learnt from the pattern of transmission in these countries remains lost on the policy makers of the developed world, who distance themselves from what their racism tells them is a 'Black problem', caused by promiscuity and backwardness. The inequitable distribution of the world's resources means that HIV hits hardest at those people to whom the most basic necessities of life are already denied. Such people are disproportionately Black, a pattern which is not confined to the economic inequalities maintained between the (over)developed nations and the third world, but is repeated in microcosm in the inner cities of the first world. It is structural and institutional racism, not innate savagery, which increases the risk of HIV infection for peoples of colour.

As always, HIV cannot be seen as a new problem. It fits into the familiar and shameful narratives of racism, so that poor Black and Latino people in the USA have disproportionately high rates of HIV infection, as they have disproportionately high rates of TB; so that Afro-Caribbean people from China to Britain have 'AIDS carrier' shouted at them along with all the other abuse; so that information is not made available to those whose cultural and religious beliefs make them 'difficult' for white people to approach; so that lesbians and gay men of colour are seldom recognized as in need of support; so that official bodies such as the blood transfusion service encourage racism by refusing blood contaminated by association with Africa; so that Black groups find it hard to get essential funding; so that white groups see racism as a 'separate issue'. A separate issue is, of course, just what it is *not*. Dr Jonathan Mann, when he was director of the World Health Organization, was clear that prejudice and discrimination, in all their forms, represented the 'third epidemic'; that the health and safety of us all depend upon the recognition that bigotry, whether directed at Blacks, gays, drug users or those already infected, is the single greatest threat to our ability to defeat AIDS.

5

Experience and expertise: uneasy collaborators in the front line

If we had been told, twenty years ago, that a new and horrible epidemic would soon be killing people in their millions in every corner of the globe, we would surely have imagined a scenario very different from the one we are witnessing today. It would have seemed unbelievable that the President of the United States would wait until *six years* into the epidemic (1987), until 25,644 Americans were *known to have died*, before even publicly recognizing the existence of a problem. It would have seemed quite incredible that in 1991, a decade into the epidemic in Britain, with officially recorded deaths of one and a half million people worldwide, and projections of tens of millions of future deaths, serious press articles and serious television and radio programmes would report the words of serious scientists denying that there is an epidemic at all, and reassuring people that they do not need to take steps to protect themselves (see, for example, Dr Peter Duesberg writing in *Science*, February 1991). How on earth do we find ourselves now in the apparently nonsensical position of endlessly debating whether there is or is not an epidemic going on, as the number of deaths grows and keeps on growing?

In answer to this question, the words of Dr Mathilde Krim, founding co-chair of the American Foundation for AIDS Research (AMFAR), are often quoted (see, for example, *AIDS DEMOgraphics*). 'This is an epidemic', she insisted, 'that could have been contained. Everything about this epidemic has been utterly predictable, from the very beginning, from the very first day. But no-one would listen.' There can be little doubt that, in simple biomedical terms, Dr Krim is quite right. We are not dealing with a contagious agent, with something which is easily transmitted by sneezing, coughing or physical contact, nor with something spread by biting insects. It is not necessary – indeed, it is not useful – to isolate infected individuals, to quarantine affected areas, to close national borders or to guard against secondary contamination from clothing, cutlery, toilet seats or doorknobs. It is simply necessary to take straightforward precautions during penetrative sex or when carrying out procedures which involve piercing the skin. Yet despite the relative simplicity of the action needed to stop the epidemic in its tracks, it shows no signs of slowing, much less halting. The reasons are, as we have seen, not medical, they are social. And the same social factors which have aided and abetted the grim progress of HIV across the planet have had an equally devastating influence on the effectiveness of the strategies we have developed to fight it.

Into the unknown

It is easy to forget the extent to which the appearance of HIV/AIDS catapulted us into the unknown. Before its sudden arrival, the developed world at least had been lulled into believing that medical science had all but conquered infectious disease. It was a tenet of medical history that the great infectious diseases were no longer a major threat to public health, and that the health care services were now able to concentrate on cancers and on the various chronic diseases and conditions, many associated with ageing, which disabled or debilitated and which tended to kill slowly and on an individual level, rather than rapidly and in huge numbers as in the bad old days of cholera, plague, typhoid or smallpox. The last major deadly epidemics had happened outside the living memory of doctors now practising, or were happening in the safely distant confines of the developing world. Distant in time and in place, the very idea of an epidemic seemed to be out of date, and the meaning of the word itself was gradually starting to shift as people spoke of 'epidemics' of non-contagious hazards such as glue-sniffing or heart disease. The structures of the medical establishment too had evolved in response to the very different set of demands now being made of them. The new structures were quite simply not designed to respond to a major outbreak of an infectious disease.

Another factor to be reckoned with is the extremely hierarchical nature of the medical profession. The NHS, Britain's largest single employer, is organized around rank and status in a way reminiscent of the army, with a great deal of power vested in those who, by reason of class, gender and/or professional ability, achieve consultant status. The power of consultants is maintained by a vast pyramid of lesser beings (junior doctors, nurses, radiographers, physiotherapists etc.), with the number of women and people of colour increasing the further down the pyramid you go. So most of the lowest-grade workers, the cleaners, laundry workers etc., are Black and/or female, while a female consultant is still very much a rarity. In addition, the various clinical specialisms have their own rank order, with high-status specialisms like neurosurgery and transplant surgery and low-status, 'Cinderella' specialisms such as genito-urinary medicine (GUM), geriatric medicine and community medicine. This internal hierarchy has real implications for patient care, and for research; high-status specialisms have traditionally tended to be high-tech and to confer 'star' status on those who practise within them, while the Cinderella specialisms are generally low-tech and regarded as pretty unexciting. Compare, for example, the public face of transplant surgery, which made an international playboy star out of Dr Christian Barnard and which still gets national news coverage, with the public image of the mental health or geriatric specialisms. Clearly, the high-profile, high-status specialisms find it much easier to attract such essentials as high-calibre staff, funding for research or publicity than the Cinderella specialisms, which have little power and attract precious little funding.

The implications of this are twofold. Firstly, the care of patients is likely to relate to the status of the clinical specialism within which their particular condition falls. A moment's reflection is enough to recognize the realities of this process; we are familiar with press reports sensationalizing the scandalous treatment of the mentally ill or the elderly within institutions established for their care, and with the idea that such people are regarded by society as 'a problem' and

On BBC 2 now, there is a programme celebrating the life and work of a world-famous playboy chiropodist - "Corns of Gold".

that we perceive the work of caring for them as doing society's 'dirty work'. The contrast with the glamorous work of the brain surgeon or the 'star' status granted the heroic transplant patient could hardly be greater!

But it is the second implication of this hierarchy which concerns us here. The fact is that the medical profession is granted an enormous amount of power in contemporary Western culture. Historians, such as Barbara Ehrenreich, Dierdre English or Michel Foucault, have pointed out that as the power of the priest waned so the power of the doctor grew. We now allow doctors to write many of the rules by which we live, and indeed to influence the law-making processes of government too (the British Medical Association has a great deal of influence at Westminster). It is now medicine (especially psychiatric medicine) rather than religion to which we turn for our guidance as to what is 'normal' and what is 'abnormal', what is wilfully deviant (and hence criminal) and what is pathological (and hence illness). It is according to medical criteria that we attempt either to punish or to cure, and it is according to medical notions of 'normality' that we live our social, sexual and emotional lives and bring up our children. The medical 'voice' speaks in our culture with enormous authority. This is not, however, true for medicine across the board. The Cinderella specialisms have greater difficulty gaining access to the public ear, and hence greater difficulty in getting their voice heard, both within the medical establishment and outside it. It was crucial for the early response to HIV/AIDS that genito-urinary medicine, the clinical area where the new condition first caused alarm, was one of the Cinderella specialisms.

Cinderella doctors, Cinderella patients

Just as there are low-status doctors, so there are low-status patients, marginalized within society and within the health care system, whose marginality tends to rub off on those working with them. These low-status patients typically include the elderly, women, those with profound intellectual impairment and the mentally ill. Racism, too, is as prevalent in the health care system as it is in any other institution.

Lesbians and gay men, who form a marginalized and profoundly stigmatized group in society generally and hence within the health care system as well, have in addition a very specific reason for mistrusting the medical profession. It is only recently that homosexuality has officially lost its label of 'illness', and the history of clinical attempts to 'cure' people of their desire and love for their own sex makes chilling reading. Whether motivated by the physical (hormone deficiency, chromosomal abnormality) or the psychological (dysfunctional parenting, unfulfilled Oedipus/Electra complex) model of homosexuality as illness, practitioners have subjected lesbians and gay men to aversion therapy, starvation, solitary confinement, drugging, electric shocks to the brain or body parts and surgical removal of parts of their brains or their genitals in an attempt to make them 'normal'. There are still medical practitioners who claim that homosexuality is 'caused' by chromosomal abnormality or by neuropsychological malfunction, despite irrefutable evidence of the flexibility and mutability of human sexual object-choice (many men, and even more women, choose to change their sexual orientation late in life, often to homosexuality after many years of successful and happy heterosexual life). It is, too, hard for lesbians and gay men to trust a profession whose members can publicly state that they 'view homosexuals with the kind of vague loathing that I view terrorists', as one British doctor did in the *General Practitioner* (cited by Simon Watney in his book *Policing Desire*). Such bigotry is not confined to the British medical establishment. On 31 August 1987, *Newsweek* revealed that a group of Soviet medical students had written to the Soviet Academy of Medical Science calling AIDS 'a noble epidemic', because, they continued, it would 'wipe out all drug addicts, homosexuals and prostitutes'. Medical professionals who thus applaud a global epidemic on the grounds that certain groups of people *should die* hardly encourage the trust of those groups whose oppression they have historically been complicit in maintaining.

If lesbians and gays are near the bottom of this hierarchy of stigma within the health care system, there is one group at the very bottom – injecting drug users. Because what they do is illegal, and because drug use is seen as a personal choice to inflict self-harm, drug users tend to be regarded with little respect by health care workers. Additionally, because illegal drug use and in particular drug addiction soaks up a lot of money, drug users who do not come into the category of the very rich (pop stars, film stars, stockbrokers) quickly become very poor. Many come from areas of great deprivation to start with (drug dependency, like most health problems, is associated with poverty and deprivation), and once they are stuck with the financial and social burden of addiction, users swiftly lose any degree of social power they may have had. The implication of this is that, whereas gay men as a social group tend to be relatively wealthy (a gay male couple generally fits into the 'DINKY' bracket – Dual Income, No Kids Yet) and hence possessed of the social power which money confers, injecting drug users as a social group tend to be extremely poor and hence profoundly disenfranchised. Additionally, gay sex has been (partially) decriminalized and gay men are no longer an illicit underground sub-group. They are, therefore, able at least in theory to stand up and demand their rights, hotly contested though these may be. Injecting drug users, because of the illicit and stigmatized nature of their drug use, are still widely regarded as not having any rights.

So when HIV/AIDS first came to light, it fitted uncannily into the very gaps which would ensure that the medical profession would find it problematic. Not only did it concern the Cinderella specialisms of community medicine, GUM and health promotion (hardly seen as within the remit of the health service at all), but also it appeared to affect two particularly stigmatized groups of health service clients, gay men and injecting drug users.

Nor was this an epidemic which gave much time for thought. Because of its characteristic lengthy period of asymptomatic infection, it was already firmly established in the populations of many nations before making its presence known, so that the identification of the virus and the classification of the new syndrome went hand in hand with the dawning realization that a global epidemic, on a scale not before witnessed in recorded history, was already under way. Additionally, as it was a sexually transmitted viral infection, the specialism called upon to deal with this frightening new phenomenon, GUM, was underfunded, underresourced and with little clout to ensure its words were heard. But perhaps most important of all was the issue of stigma, and the extent to which medical researchers, policy makers and care givers allowed their prejudice against marginalized groups to warp their professional judgement. It is sobering to recognize that the supposed neutrality of scientific medicine has been revealed by the events of the early 1980s to be nothing more than a pious sham. Dubbing the new syndrome Gay-Related Immune Deficiency (GRID), researchers busied themselves looking for factors *in the gay lifestyle* which could lead to this kind of damage, speculating that it was 'fast track living' which so ravaged the immune system. It is only when we compare this approach with the way in which Legionnaires' Disease was handled that the strangeness of assuming that the roots of a new and devastating disease lie in a way of life rather than in an external pathogen is revealed. Obviously, it would be absurd to suggest that something in the *lifestyle* of members of the American Legion was responsible for their illness. Yet so clearly is 'homosexuality' pathologized in mainstream medical thinking that this approach did not seem absurd at all when applied to gay men.

Accounts of early attempts to make some sort of logical sense out of the bewildering symptoms of the new syndrome read alarmingly like magic. It is hard to believe that the mighty and inexorable logic of modern biomedicine could come up with something as frankly childlike as the American '4 Hs' model of 1981-2, which postulated (in direct contradiction of the evidence as it existed even then) that heroin addicts, homosexuals, Haitians and haemophiliacs were 'risk groups' for this sickness. (Strange that no-one should have rocked medical science with the discovery that heterosexual, too, begins with 'H'!) Such playing with words smacks more of superstition and numerology than of scientific rationality, yet the '4 Hs' model was accorded widespread credibility.

Early responses

Two features characterize the early response to HIV/AIDS in the USA and Britain. The first is the consciousness that, faced with an already well-established epidemic, the only available option was fire-fighting, working reactively rather than proactively, with everything happening at once. The second is the development of 'deviant' expertise.

Fire-fighting

HIV/AIDS is a public health problem on a massive scale. It is also an educational problem on a massive scale. Everyone alive needs information, we all need different information and we all need information appropriately targeted and in language we are familiar with. Those already infected need to be informed about medical developments, complementary health care strategies, nutrition, stress management, any health problems related to ownership of specific pet animals etc., in order to prolong survival time and maximize quality of life. They also need to know how to prevent transmission of HIV to those close to them, especially sexual partners, fellow drug users or children. So all that information needs to be researched, developed and disseminated to those who need it. Additionally, people with HIV and/or AIDS need information about rights and benefits, wills and inheritance, insurance, employment, adoption, fostering and respite care for children, so that they may plan their lives accordingly. So laws need to be drawn up and carried through Parliament, legal precedents must be established, advice and caring agencies must be briefed and procedures for insurance, benefit claims etc. must be negotiated.

Those not known to be infected need to know how to protect themselves and those close to them from infection, including safer sex and drug use techniques (see appendices 1 and 2). Those not known to be infected, but responsible for the care of, or simply close to, those who are, need information about prevention of transmission, appropriate care guidelines, access to support and counselling, as well as a sensitive awareness of the stigma associated with AIDS. Those responsible for educating others in schools, colleges, universities, adult education etc. need to understand their own responsibility to pass on accurate information about HIV and AIDS and for challenging misinformation and prejudice. They need to know what to teach about the epidemic and how to teach it to their client group. Educational materials need to be developed, tested, disseminated and evaluated for children, young adults, people with learning difficulties, the deaf and/or visually handicapped, people with a range of disabilities, adults, different religious and ethnic groups, those whose mother tongue is not English and, of course, every possible combination of all these.

Those whose work brings them into contact with the public, or who work with colleagues, need accurate and reliable information about HIV/AIDS health and safety issues, especially in relation to First Aid. First Aiders and health care workers need specific training which may have to cover everything from safe disposal of used sharps to mouth-to-mouth resuscitation. General practitioners in particular need training in the recognition of early symptoms of HIV infection (especially in those who do not fit the 'at risk' stereotypes), as well as in the practical and social implications of taking an HIV antibody test, the continuing care of someone with HIV and/or AIDS and supporting the families of those who are infected or ill. Those who work with people who are known to have HIV or AIDS need training in counselling skills as well as clinical care, and in the

social implications for those touched by such a stigmatizing condition. Policy makers need to be trained to identify and respond
appropriately to the policy implications which HIV/AIDS has for
areas such as education, health care, housing, benefits, economics,
human rights, employment, social work etc. etc.

Faced with such an overwhelming public education agenda on
top of the urgent need to find out how best to care for people sick
with AIDS-related illnesses, to identify the cause of AIDS and
research possible cures and vaccines, the only possible response
was fire-fighting, a chaotic series of ad hoc responses to each
situation as it arose. This lent a sense of urgency and confusion to
AIDS work in the early days of the epidemic, a sense which has
become numbed through familiarity rather than left behind, as we
are in no way 'on top of' the epidemic.

'Deviant' expertise

The second feature which was so startling at the beginning of the
epidemic was that the entire concept of medical expertise was
momentarily stood on its head, as the communities most affected by
the new syndrome rapidly developed an extraordinarily wide range
of survival skills while the customary 'experts' stalled. It was quite
clear that this was a problem which could not be satisfactorily dealt
with within existing structures. It was equally clear that the political
will to recognize the existence of a problem, let alone to deal with
it, was not there. Rendered smug and uncaring by a deeply ingrained
homophobia, the establishment was dragging its heels while the
death toll mounted. So it was left to the gay community, first in the
USA and soon after in Britain and the rest of Europe, to devise
strategies for fighting this new and terrifying unknown killer.

The response of the American gay community was not automatic.
Writers such as Randy Schultz, in *And the Band Played On*, and Larry
Kramer, in *Reports from the Holocaust*, have documented the initial
resistance of gay men to the idea that there was a risk, and that
community activism was essential if the carnage was to be slowed. In
1981, six gay men met to discuss their fears about what then appeared
to be an epidemic of Kaposi's sarcoma (see pp. 5–6). From this initial

meeting Gay Men's Health Crisis (GMHC) was born, now the longest-lived AIDS organization in the world, and set up entirely through fund-raising in the gay community. In 1983 Larry Kramer published an article he headlined '1,112 and Counting' in the gay community paper *New York Native.* The opening words of the article read, 'If this article doesn't scare the shit out of you, we're in real trouble. If this article doesn't rouse you to anger, fury, rage and action, gay men may have no future on this earth. Our continued existence depends on just how angry you can get.' Kramer was convinced that civil disobedience was the only way to get the US establishment to take notice of AIDS, something that GMHC was not prepared to endorse. Rather than taking on the major political struggle of getting the state to abide by its responsibilities *vis-à-vis* AIDS, the greater part of the gay community response was to provide *directly* those services which were not being provided by the state. And it was in the process of developing these services that the gay community became the new 'experts' of the epidemic. With the example of the organization and activism of two decades of feminist health campaigning, the gay community set about identifying and meeting their own needs.

Thus, even before HIV was identified as the causative agent for AIDS, safer sex guidelines were being developed by gay men in the USA. In 1983 a group of gay men, including PWAs, published a 40-page booklet of safer sex guidelines, 'How to Have Sex in an Epidemic', which still stands as the best of its kind today. Safer sex was developed by the gay community as a political response to an epidemic which the rest of the world seemed intent on ignoring. Gay men rapidly became the acknowledged 'experts' on health promotion, transmission prevention and the psycho-social aspects of the epidemic itself, and of the changes in sexual behaviour it necessitated. Gay physicians and community workers found their community experience becoming valuable expertise. The safe sex information developed in the States was disseminated through the grapevine of gay community publications around the world, meeting resistance, confiscation and legal action from heterosexual agencies and government bodies on its life-saving way. In Britain, HM Customs and Excise impounded copies of American gay magazines and newspapers as obscene, and police raiding Gay's The Word, the

London community bookshop, made off with HIV/AIDS educational material along with novels and magazines.

The gay community response has been on many levels, from instituting the network of 'buddies' – volunteers who befriend PWAs and offer support with day-to-day tasks like shopping – to devising often imaginative health promotion initiatives. The contrast between the methods developed by this community, a group of people who are, by and large, open and uninhibited about all things sexual, and the wider heterosexual community is striking. In 1988, for example, the newly elected Miss America wanted to spend some of her year in office working for AIDS education; this idea was greeted with firm disapproval and she was prevented from carrying it out. In total contrast, the groups who sponsor the gay men's equivalent, the annual 'Mr Leather' contest, have made it a condition of winning that Mr Leather should spend his year in office doing just that. The comparison makes the tabloid accusations of gay men's 'irresponsibility' ring particularly hollow.

Uptight, outasight and not promoting health

Both in the USA and in Britain, the dawning recognition of the nature and seriousness of the epidemic came at a difficult and embarrassing historical moment. In both countries the new right was politically committed to a symbolic crusade against 'permissiveness', a rigorously imposed reign of discipline (depicted as both fiscal and moral) to root out what was seen as the left-over radicalism of the 1960s and replace it with the 'new' morality. The message was overtly Christian, fundamentalist in tone, and characterized by a sentimental and romantic harking back to times past, specifically to a (misrepresented) version of 'Victorian values'. A distinguishing characteristic of this ideology was the concerned anxiety directed at the family. 'A nation of free people', declared the then Prime Minister Margaret Thatcher in May 1988, 'will only continue to be great if family life continues and the structure of that nation is a family one.' The notion of the family constructed within and by this ideology is a very specific one, imagined as essentially good, essentially normal and essentially *moral* within the terms of a narrow, received moralism; and in the hands of the New Right it became, in Salman Rushdie's phrase, 'totemized'. The political determination to defend the family from the frankly demonized forces of promiscuity and homosexuality allowed the British and American right-wing governments to take upon themselves a mandate for state and legislative intervention in people's intimate sexual and emotional lives to an extent not witnessed since the Third Reich.

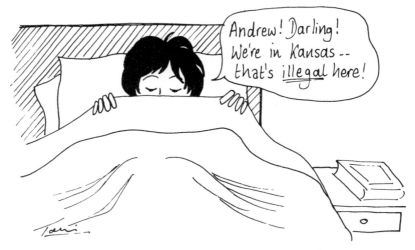

Children were, at all costs, to be protected from the bogeymen of the anxious and fevered new right imagination. In the USA, the 1987 Helms amendment attempted to make it illegal for lesbians and gay men to teach in schools, while in Britain the education system was tied to the promotion of a particular political ideology as never before. In a chilling speech at the 1987 Tory Party conference, Thatcher asserted that 'Children who need to be taught to respect traditional moral values are being taught that they have an inalienable right to be gay.' In other words, sexual and emotional relationships, widely regarded as 'private' and certainly *not* as the business of the state, are not a matter of personal choice any longer. None of us has the 'inalienable right' to choose how we express our most intimate feelings, nor with whom.

Fired by the belief that sexuality was a force which should be harnessed to the good of the nation, a new doctrine on sex education was developed and implemented. Despite teachers and Her Majesty's Inspectorate consistently declaring that more and better sex education in schools was urgently needed, and despite research findings which showed that the majority of parents were rather anxious that schools *should* provide comprehensive sex education for their children (see, for example, Isobel Allen's report, *Education in Sex and Personal Relationships*, for the Policy Studies Institute), new measures were instituted whereby sex education was handed over, lock, stock and barrel, to school governors. It was left to the discretion of governors in individual schools to decide whether or not sex education should take place in their school. Where a decision was taken that sex education should take place, it was the responsibility of governors to draw up and make public a formal sex education policy.

Homosexuality was deployed very successfully by the New Right in the attempt to gain public support for their ideological onslaught. A series of press-incited mini-panics about lesbian and gay sex being 'taught' in schools culminated in the drafting of Section 28 of the 1988 Local Government Act, which states that: '(1) A local authority shall not: (a) intentionally promote homosexuality or publish material with the intention of promoting homosexuality; (b) promote the teaching in any maintained school of the acceptability of homosexuality as a pretended family relationship.' Although the government was subsequently obliged to send out a circular to all schools explaining that the new law did not apply to them (schools do not come within the remit of this Act), research, such as that reported in the University of Birmingham Cultural Studies Group publication *Off Centre*, indicates that Section 28 has had a powerful negative effect on schools and colleges alike, to the detriment of activities as diverse as Theatre in Education performances, book buying in school libraries and equal opportunities work.

In this fearful and rigid climate, HIV/AIDS work poses peculiar difficulties.

Uneasy bedfellows: the early days of the epidemic in Britain

When it came to promoting public health and protecting its subjects from an epidemic which was transmitted sexually or by sharing drug-injecting equipment, and which affected large numbers of gay men, the establishment in Britain had already firmly tied its own hands. The dilemma was a painful and farcical one. The dictates of infection control, faced with a lethal new epidemic, demanded that explicit and detailed information about sexual and drug-injecting practices be made available to everyone, and that support should be given to enable people to put into practice a set of potentially painful changes in their personal lives. The dictates of right-wing familial ideology demanded that behaviours previously labelled as deviant, dangerous and politically destabilizing (namely, homosexuality, promiscuity and illegal drug use) should be marginalized, stigmatized and punished. The only sexual behaviour to be tolerated was heterosexual, strictly monogamous and sanctioned by (preferably life-long) marriage. Young people had to be *taught* these things. Additionally, the administration was beset by the unlikely notion that merely to mention something 'bad' was tantamount to promoting it. It was as though, faced with the question of how to (or rather, whether to) represent behaviours seen as deviant, politicians had not progressed beyond the somewhat simplistic analytical model, 'monkey see – monkey do'.

Hedged about by self-made obstacles, and loath to be seen to be reneging on its ideological commitments, the administration was forced into a ludicrous compromise. The first national AIDS campaign resorted to evasiveness on a staggering scale, presenting a bemused public with alarming images of a geological nature stolen from cheap B movies, capped by crashing tombstones and bathed in sepulchral gloom. This was swiftly followed up by a truly incisive campaign in 1987 urging us all not to die of ignorance, a sage piece of advice which, given the inadequacy and general scarcity of information on offer, seemed to aspire to the heights of Zen enlightenment. It was far more likely that the British public would tune in to the sound of one hand clapping than that we would be able to get our hands on the information we needed to prevent us dying of government-sponsored ignorance.

Meanwhile, working far away from the dry ice and monumental masonry, the gay community was taking HIV/AIDS on board, as it had done in the States. In 1983 the friends of Terrence Higgins, one of the first gay men to die with AIDS in Britain, found themselves appalled by the lack of care and support available to him during his illness and death. They sought and received help from the Greater London Council and the Health Education Council, and held a conference in the Conway Hall in London, inviting a speaker from the AIDS organization in Boston. From this the Terrence Higgins Trust (THT) was born. Health education and information provision was the first aim, and the Trust set about producing AIDS education leaflets and materials, initially for gay men but very quickly for a much wider audience. For two years, funding came entirely from fund-raising in the gay community, while the Trust lobbied the government for a response to the epidemic. On 14 February 1984 (an auspicious date if ever there was one!) a telephone help line was set up, and in September 1985 a government grant of £35,000 was received to fund this and to produce more leaflets. At the time, the THT was the only thing available for people affected by or worried about AIDS, and was barely able to cope with the demand for information. It was not only individual members of the public who came to rely on the Trust for information, it was the press, media and government bodies. The reversal of expertise which had happened in the States was repeated in Britain.

For the government, the existence of the THT was the only possible way out of the ideological corner they had painted themselves into. Not only was the gay community providing money for the initiatives which should by rights have been government funded, but the Trust was able and willing to undertake essential health education work with and for gay men, work which the government was, for political reasons, extremely unwilling to be seen to be doing. In 1983, the same year as the Conway Hall conference, the Medical Research Council (MRC) set up a working party on AIDS, and in January 1985 the government set up the Expert Advisory Group on AIDS (EAGA). Both proved slow and unsatisfactory. The overt agenda was that, now it was known that AIDS did not 'just' affect gay men, public action was necessary. This took the form of implementing the Public Health and Control of Diseases Act (1984), which mandated the enforced hospitalization and, if necessary, detention of PWAs (a measure with little epidemiological justification), and setting up a blood screening programme (too late to prevent the infection with HIV of thousands of haemophiliacs).

On not putting your money where your mouth is

The government response to AIDS was largely shaped by the political necessity of being seen to do something for the general public (read, 'heterosexuals') while continuing to insist on the deviant status of homosexuality, extramarital sex and injecting drug use, and distancing itself from anything which appeared to 'condone' such behaviours, such as needle exchange schemes or distributing condoms in prisons. It needed to keep political control of the AIDS agenda, and this need took clear precedence over the responsibility to fight the spread of this epidemic and to safeguard the health of its subjects. Thus in January 1987 the government commissioned the all-party Social Services Committee to investigate the progress of the epidemic and the provision of care in the UK, but proceeded to delay its response to the Committee's (highly critical) final report by a year, and to ignore its recommendations. Similarly, the autonomous Health Education Council (which had been a quite outspoken critic of government health policy in general, and AIDS policy in particular) was disbanded in 1986 and replaced by a restructured body, the Health Education Authority, which was made responsible for a significant AIDS budget, but simultaneously brought within the structure of the health service, and made directly accountable to Westminster.

Given the political nature of the government response to AIDS, it is hard to see how community organizations like the Terrence Higgins Trust could hope to get financial backing from central government without sacrifices. As Zoe Schramm-Evans points out in her historical account of one year of the epidemic in l *Responses to AIDS: 1986–1987*, the attitude of the administra......... the day to THT becomes clear when comparing the total government funding of £466,000 which the Trust received up to autumn 1987 with the ex gratia payment of £10 million given to the Haemophilia Society to set up a trust fund for HIV+ haemophiliacs. The problems attendant on trying to co-operate with a basically hostile government soon became all too clear. Early in 1987 the infamous 'Don't Die of Ignorance' leaflet was delivered to every household in the land. Although the Trust had not been consulted during the drawing up of this campaign, their telephone number appeared in the leaflet (along with that of London Lesbian and Gay Switchboard), resulting in a deluge of calls from panic-stricken callers which all but swamped them. No additional funding or support was made available to organizations struggling to deal with this response. Problems became desperate later that year, as the overburdened accounting system at THT collapsed, while government funds which had been promised were held up by the general election, and were, when eventually received, £250,000 less than agreed.

The two sides to community action

Despite the headaches involved in attempting to work in co-operation with central government, the THT is now the largest AIDS service organization in Britain, providing a telephone help line, a counselling service, training and education, welfare and legal advice, a hardship fund for PWAs, a buddying network and a range of well-produced AIDS educational material including posters, packs and leaflets. And AIDS support organizations have mushroomed. Body Positive, a support network of and for people with HIV infection and/or AIDS, now has thirty branches nationally, produces a national fortnightly free newsletter and has a drop-in centre in London. It includes women's and a young people's support groups, and sends speakers to conferences, schools and workshops. It is sobering to compare the £40,000 annual grant to Body Positive *nationally* (used as small grants to help people in hardship) with the £400,000 budget of New York Body Positive after one year of operation. Even more sobering is the position of Positively Women, an organization set up by Caroline Guiness when she was diagnosed HIV+ and found a complete lack of appropriate support for women. Four women now run a national organization, virtually unfunded, struggling to provide services for HIV+ women while having to negotiate a maze of organizational work, fund-raise and provide speakers for radio and television programmes, schools, newspaper and magazine interviews and conferences.

As it has become obvious that the government is not going to allocate resources to meeting the needs which different groups may have for AIDS-related education and support, the voluntary sector has tended to organize around very specific issues. Thus, Black HIV/AIDS Network (BHAN) was set up in October 1988 with no funding, and continues the struggle to identify and meet the needs of the Black communities. The Mildmay Mission and London Lighthouse provide volunteer nursing and residential care to PWAs, including a hospice facility, while the Mildmay is initiating specialist nurse training courses and finding ways to integrate HIV/AIDS training into existing nurse training programmes. AIDS Ahead, based in Carlisle, was set up in 1987 with help from the Terrence Higgins Trust to produce educational materials for people who are deaf and hard of hearing, while Immunity Legal Centre, set up by concerned volunteers with legal training, exists to provide advice and support on the legal aspects of HIV infection, and liaises with local hospitals. Outside London, local voluntary AIDS support organizations such as the Aled Richards Trust in Bristol and OXAIDS in Oxford, or education projects such as the Sheffield AIDS Education Project and the Liverpool HIV/AIDS Team, work to provide a range of services, with varying degrees of support from their local authorities. Such groups operate under terrific strain. Not only do they have to stretch inadequate budgets to cover ever-increasing need, they have to do so in an area where there is still widespread public ignorance and prejudice. AIDS is not an easy area to work in, even for health professionals. When the Royal College of Nurses published guidelines for nursing PWAs, they received four or five anonymous hate phone calls per night on the telephone answering machine for months. In the face of such pointless and stubborn hostility, it is hard to maintain a sense of optimism and purpose.

The stresses of volunteering

The vast majority of work in the provision of services to people affected by HIV/AIDS (other than medical care) goes on in the voluntary sector. Typically, an organization will manage to get funding (often temporary) to pay one or two full-time workers, and will have a complement of volunteers, many with HIV themselves, giving as much time as they are able in return for expenses (bus fares etc.) and job satisfaction. There are structural problems built in to this model. Volunteers tend not to remain with any organization indefinitely; two years is about average, and this time tends to be shorter working in an intense and stressful area such as HIV/AIDS. Volunteer 'burn-out' is common, and strategies (such as proper co-ordination, supervision and support) must be evolved to prevent this. The rapid turnover of essential workers means that volunteer recruitment, training, supervision and management are an on-going process. There is never a point at which an organization can say, 'OK, we've got the staff, now let's do the work.'

Another major problem lies in the never-ending stream of thankless administrative tasks which must be carried out efficiently if the organization is to survive. Funding applications must be completed (often annually) and returned to funding bodies on time, together with any additional documentation in support of the application. In a climate where burgeoning numbers of worthy causes are competing for restricted resources, research into alternative or additional sources of income must be on-going. Fund-raising activities must be organized, both to supplement income and to keep the organization in the public eye locally. Volunteer recruitment, especially in a small area, is often problematic, as new people must be sought from further afield as the 'pool' of available volunteers begins to dry up. Information about the medical and social aspects of HIV/AIDS changes rapidly, and this must be kept track of. Links with other organizations must be established and maintained, letters answered, enquiries settled, negative publicity handled tactfully and positive publicity capitalized upon skilfully. Good relations must be established with local press and media, questions relating to national and local issues must be fielded. Accounts must be kept, often involving quite substantial sums of money, and annual auditing arranged to the satisfaction of funding bodies. Evaluation must be carried out, annual reports written, a management committee appointed and its meetings regularly attended.

Most people who get involved in work with HIV/AIDS, as with any other kind of voluntary work, do so because they want to do something to help. They are unlikely to want to spend hours of their free time going through the books or chasing up funding applications. Additionally, much essential administrative work demands continuity. It is unimpressive if the local director of social services can never get to speak to the same person twice when ringing to discuss future funding arrangements! So organizations are presented with a problem. In order to work with HIV/AIDS effectively, you need commitment, energy and sensitivity, especially in the areas of sexuality and drug use. In order to be an effective administrator, you may need quite different qualities – a good head for figures, a way with words, shrewdness and toughness – qualities which are not often found hand in hand with the tact and sensitivity of a good HIV/AIDS worker. All too often the 'real' work of the organization, the grass-roots, front-line work of meeting need, takes up all the energy of the workers, with the result that the mundane but essential administrative work gets neglected. Similarly, if an organization manages to attract funding for two workers, it is easy to understand the reluctance to appoint one co-ordinator of volunteers and one administrator, leaving the 'real' work to the volunteers.

Because the AIDS epidemic is an emergency, and because the voluntary sector of what Cindy Patton calls the 'AIDS industry' (see her chapter in Erica Carter and Simon Watney's book *Taking Liberties*) was forced to grow so fast to cope, real problems arose, with a desperate shortage of experienced administrators to manage the mushrooming swarm of organizations, often for risible wages compared to what was on offer in business or industry. The people who wanted to work with HIV/AIDS wanted to help PWAs; they wanted to be buddies, to be on the end of the telephone help lines, to counsel and support the newly diagnosed, partners and the bereaved. Many non-statutory AIDS support organizations, including major ones such as the Terrence Higgins Trust and the Sussex AIDS Trust, have run into big administrative problems, and have been forced to devote valuable time, energy and money to rescue operations. Meanwhile, the large government budget allocated to HIV/AIDS (£20 million in 1986) does not reach the non-statutory organizations who are doing most of the grass-roots work, but is channelled into local health authority budgets, where it has all too often been used by some authorities (see articles in *The Pink Paper* during January and February 1992) in creative accounting to set against budget deficits.

There is an interesting footnote to AIDS volunteering, as yet again the epidemic shows up in sharp relief the inequitable structures in our society. For, while 50 per cent of volunteer 'buddies' are women, and the rest mostly gay men, almost none are white heterosexual men. Yet, as writer Simon Watney points out in his introduction to *Taking Liberties*, it is largely white heterosexual men who earn the big money associated with HIV/AIDS, as consultants, medical researchers, drug company directors, journalists, television producers etc.

When does co-operation become collusion?

There is a growing lobby in the 'AIDS community' which insists that it has been a grave mistake for gay men to respond to the AIDS crisis in the way they have. By setting up such a large and comprehensive voluntary sector to identify and meet the needs of communities affected by HIV, they argue, unique political opportunities have been lost. From this perspective, the hard work of volunteers, drawn mainly from those for whom HIV and AIDS are of central personal significance, simply colludes with and reinforces the oppressive and negligent behaviour of central government and of a bigoted and reactionary sector of society. There are important ways in which this criticism is undoubtedly accurate.

Firstly, those working in the voluntary sector generally need no convincing that AIDS is an issue for them. Some are themselves HIV+ or living with AIDS, others are lovers, family members or friends of people who are infected or sick or who have died. Yet others are members of communities and social groups for whom HIV and AIDS have a particular significance: the gay community, struggling to resist scapegoating and opprobrium at the same time as seeing too many friends and lovers become ill and die; Black and minority ethnic communities forced to recognize that their needs for AIDS education care and support are not recognized by the establishment; women who have always borne the burden of caring for the sick while getting little support and care when sick themselves, and for whom HIV/AIDS represents another chapter in the same old story of neglect and abuse. It can be argued that it is heterosexual men who have, as a group, shown most resistance to AIDS education messages, who have proved most reluctant to change their behaviour and to take responsibility for safer sex, and who have consistently put the health of women and of gay men at risk by the intransigence of their denial. When AIDS is 'taken care of' by means of a self-selected voluntary workforce, heterosexual men (and others still stuck in a state of denial) are allowed to get away with it, to remain wilfully ignorant of the true nature and extent of the epidemic, to repeat over and over again the tired old lies that AIDS is for queers and junkies but not for them. By a combination of circumstances, AIDS is being socially ghettoized. Within the medical industry, it is increasingly accruing to itself a conglomeration of specialisms and becoming structurally isolated from the mainstream. Within society generally, an 'AIDS community' has grown up, serving to insulate the wider public from the medical and social realities of the syndrome.

An additional implication of our dependence on the non-statutory sector is that the state, too, is allowed to 'get away with it'. This has particularly grave political consequences for lesbians and gay men, and for the current crisis in health care policy more generally. Voluntary work and the charitable sector in particular have always posed political dilemmas with relation to the welfare state. Vital though it clearly is to lobby on behalf of people in need, it is equally vital to prevent the state offloading the business of providing services on to volunteers and washing its hands of its responsibilities. In the case of AIDS this is especially important. Gay men pay national insurance, income tax and local government charges (whatever these are called at one time or another!); they contribute their labour and their spending power to the economy. They are entitled as of right to full and appropriate health care, free at the point of receipt, and to all other benefits of the welfare state. They are entitled to have their interests represented in Parliament, and to their rightful share of the benefits and services provided by national and local government. What has in fact happened in relation to HIV/ AIDS is that national government has, by allocating funds to organizations such as the Terrence Higgins Trust, been able to offload its responsibilities towards gay men (especially with regard to health education) while continuing to attack homosexuality and homosexuals actively in public. It is chilling to reflect that, as the extent of the epidemic became clear, anti-homosexual legislation was being debated in the House of Commons. Many would argue that, by taking upon itself the task of providing AIDS-related services to gay men, the gay community is colluding with the establishment homophobia which denies them the most basic rights.

It is out of this perspective that the phenomenon of AIDS activism was born. Learning from the non-violent direct action campaigns of the women's peace movement and of ecological organizations such as Greenpeace, which had so successfully captured the public imagination, direct action AIDS campaigning began. Larry Kramer, the public-spirited and outspoken gadfly of the US gay community, saw quite clearly that 'most of Gay Men's Health Crisis' efforts are devoted to providing services the city [New York] should be providing', and called an open meeting at the New York Lesbian and Gay Community Centre early in 1987. From this meeting, documented in Kramer's book *Reports from the Holocaust*, ACTUP (AIDS Coalition To Unleash Power) was born. The goal of the group, according to Kramer, was 'to demonstrate our anger and frustration at this intolerable situation, create a critical mass of

118 Antibody politic: AIDS and society

informed public opinion and influence our leaders to take constructive action'. Stressing always their rejection of the symbolic disempowerment of PWAs by labelling them 'patients', 'victims' or 'sufferers', and replacing action on behalf of PWAs by organizing *with* PWAs (who made up a significant segment of ACTUP's membership), the new group launched a campaign of civil disobedience and symbolic protest. Demonstrations demanded changes in drugs trial procedures and increased funding for AIDS treatment research, and ACTUP attracted important media attention to an issue which had threatened to become 'stale'. A nerve had clearly been touched; ACTUP chapters sprang up in major cities throughout the States, and in the UK. ACTUP acts as the political conscience of AIDS work, zapping events which it sees as colluding with heterosexist oppression and demonstrating in demand of a proper and adequate statutory response to the epidemic. In some areas (including, in the UK, London) women have set up separate chapters of ACTUP in order to draw attention to the often neglected issues facing women with HIV/AIDS.

Re-gaying AIDS? Dilemmas of identity

There is another powerful contradiction at work for gay men concerned about HIV/AIDS. How should we characterize the relationship between gay men and the epidemic? Of course it is crucial to destroy the oppressive and dangerous myth that AIDS is (a) limited to gay men, (b) the punishment for or just deserts of deviant sexual behaviour or (c) caused by, or introduced to 'the general public' by, gay men. Yet it is also essential to recognize the devastation and pain which have been visited upon the gay community and to respect and honour the solidarity and determination with which large numbers of gay men have taken responsibility for their own *and often for heterosexuals as well.*

For those working in HIV/AIDS who are not gay men, there is another set of problems. The neglect and oppression of people of colour, women, the elderly, people with disabilities and working-class people are as prevalent among gay men as among many other social groups, and there are those who feel that the AIDS agenda, having been seized by gay men in the early days in order for them to survive, has never been sufficiently opened out to take on the needs of other groups. On the other hand, there are those gay men who argue that the professionalization of AIDS has resulted in gay issues being marginalized once more. Indeed, in 1990 a European conference held in Amsterdam was called 'Re-gaying AIDS'.

There is probably truth in both accounts. For gay men, the inversion of expertise in the early days of the epidemic led to an unfamiliar sense of being important, of being heard, of having unaccustomed power. There was also the heady experience of being part of an exclusive community drawn close together to face an emergency. Irredeemably ghastly as this epidemic has been for gay men, there have been undoubted benefits for the sense of community and of group identity. And yet, gay men are not 'political' in the way that the women's movement, for example, is political. Gay men are unused to handling issues such as race, disability and class, familiar political issues which have at one time or another rocked the women's movement. Gay men also, as they emerged from their closets to take their place in the fight against AIDS, turned out to be well represented in powerful positions in academia, in the establishment, in the NHS, in publishing, and have been well placed to foreground (quite rightly) their own issues and concerns. Other marginalized groups, women, disabled people and people of colour, represent the most powerless and disenfranchised groups in society, something which is clearly reflected in the desperate lack of attention given to their HIV/AIDS-related needs. It is clear that, rather than competing for ownership of the AIDS agenda, what is needed is a strong and politically acute alliance, a recognition of the common root of many oppressions, and the determination to move towards broadly based and inclusive theoretical and working practices. As we have seen, all the oppressions, all the 'isms' are reinforced by the current social response to AIDS, and in turn they all aid and abet the epidemic in its global spread. It is only by fighting all the 'isms' on a united front that a successful strategy to fight the epidemic can ever be devised and carried through.

6

Conclusion: into the future

It is tempting, faced with the meaningless havoc wrought by a virus, to fall back on statistics to give us some sense of control, some notion that we can plan for the future with a degree of confidence. Unfortunately, that is perhaps the thing most difficult to do with HIV/AIDS. It is very hard for a culture accustomed to the magic which can be worked by numbers to grasp the full implications of a virus which can have a latency period of ten or twelve years and which may cause no recognizable symptoms for the whole of that time. It is very hard to understand the implications of our realization that human immunodeficiency virus has probably been around since the 1950s. We have to accept that statistics on the extent of the epidemic are likely to be inaccurate, and that accurate predictions of the numbers likely to fall sick in the future are quite simply an impossibility. Yet the statistics which we do have, limited though they are, make chilling reading.

As I write this in the last days in 1991, the number of *recorded* individuals who have tested positive for antibodies to HIV in the UK has reached 16,248. Given that this represents those who have sufficient reason to believe themselves at risk to have come forward for testing, it is clear that this probably represents a fraction of those actually infected. There have been 5,065 *recorded* cases of AIDS up to the end of November (again, this is likely to be an underestimate), of whom 3,156 are known to have died already. At the end of June 1991, the number of recorded AIDS cases was 4,758, of whom 2,759 had died. In five months we have seen an increase of almost 7 per cent in the number of those with AIDS, and we have lost 397 people. Of the thirty countries in Europe, the UK ranks fifth highest for numbers of people with AIDS, with a caseload greater than that of thirty-two African countries.

It is often said that the epidemic in the United Kingdom tends to repeat the pattern in the United States, with a time lag of three to five years. In the USA, the Public Health Service estimates that one to one and a half million people are HIV infected. The number of *reported* cases of AIDS passed the 100,000 mark as long ago as August 1989. AIDS is now the commonest cause of death for women of childbearing age in New York and many other major US cities. It is the commonest cause of death among the prison population in the USA, and one study carried out in 1988 showed that one fifth of all women entering New York State prison system were HIV+. The epidemic is touching everyone. The New York City Health Department estimates that by 1995 there will be 20,000 'AIDS orphans' (uninfected babies and children who have lost both parents to AIDS), with many thousands of HIV+ babies and children similarly orphaned. The Panos Institute predicts that there will be at least 75,000 and probably as many as 85,000 uninfected children orphaned by AIDS in NYC by the end of the decade. The rate of *recorded* AIDS deaths in the US population is currently around 470 per million, ten times higher than in the UK. There is as yet nothing to give cause for optimism that what has happened in New York will not be repeated in London, Glasgow, Belfast, Bristol or Liverpool.

I do not believe that, as a society, we have begun to get to grips with what the HIV epidemic means. There is still a widespread complacency, especially among heterosexuals, that medical science is somehow dealing with it. We seem to be waiting expectantly for *Horizon* or *World in Action* to tell us that the miracle has happened, that a vaccine has been developed or a cure discovered. We still cling to the vague hope that the epidemic will burn itself out, that the virus will mutate and become harmless, that our own sexual behaviour does not count or that we are rich enough or educated enough or chaste enough or old enough not to have to worry. We are kidding ourselves. HIV is not going to go away, it is here to stay. It is as much a part of our lives as other 'new' diseases (like rheumatoid arthritis, unknown before the Industrial Revolution, with us still, and affecting millions in the UK at some time in their lives). If it does not affect us directly, what about our families, our children, our nephews and nieces, our grandchildren, our friends, colleagues, students, employees or neighbours? The issues, as we have seen, are not simply medical ones. The political, social and policy implications are vast. So, what might the future hold? What possibilities should we be thinking about now?

Implications for health care

There is much optimistic talk of a possible vaccine against HIV infection, or of treatment to limit the harm done by the virus once an individual is infected. Some accounts suggest that we will have a useable vaccine by 1995, though there are less optimistic suggestions that the end of the decade is a more likely date. In some senses, it matters little whether a vaccine is developed sooner rather than later. Vaccination is far from a magic wand, especially when used against something as mutable as a virus. True, an international vaccination programme has succeeded in eliminating smallpox, but smallpox differs from HIV in many significant ways, not least of which is that it is caused by a bacillus, not a virus. Medical science has, to date, had far more success with bacilli than with viruses. Additionally, it is clear that in order for a vaccine to eradicate HIV, the entire population of the world would probably have to be vaccinated, an unimaginably costly operation and one which presents enormous practical difficulties. Most importantly, a vaccine only means something to those who are as yet uninfected; it has nothing to offer the estimated millions who already have the virus. In this context it is perhaps pertinent to note, as British AIDS commentator Simon Watney reminds us in *Policing Desire,* that 'every penny of the £40.5 million that the Medical Research Council has received for medical research has gone to the development of a vaccine for the uninfected, while none has gone to the development of clinical trials for potential treatment drugs. People living with HIV and AIDS have simply been written off in their entirety.'

Although the medical establishment in the UK has ignored the need to develop therapies for those already antibody positive or ill with HIV diseases, such is not the case worldwide, and there is talk of HIV infection becoming a 'manageable' condition in the not too distant future, rather as diabetes is today. In the (over)developed world now, people testing positive for antibodies to HIV are offered a range of experimental prophylactic and therapeutic treatments. Prophylactic drugs, like the anti-viral agent zidovudine (AZT), appear useful in delaying the onset of symptoms and in prolonging survival time for people with HIV, although such drugs are very powerful, and side effects can be unpleasant and dangerous. Therapeutic drugs treat the various opportunistic infections associated with HIV/AIDS. There are, however, many qualifiers to bear in mind. In order to receive treatment you have to have the good fortune to live in a country where the treatments are available and where it is legal to prescribe them (many are still experimental and have not passed the necessary clinical safety trials demanded by, for example, the US Food and Drug Administration). They are expensive (AZT costs around $10,000 per year for one patient), so unless you live in a country with free health care, or are wealthy enough to afford comprehensive private health care insurance, you probably will not get access to them. One way to get access to potentially life-saving experimental drugs is to join trial programmes as a guinea pig, something which is being increasingly done by PWAs in the States. Yet women, for example, are banned from such programmes, because it is feared that expensive litigation might result from (potential) harm caused to (potential) foetuses by experimental drugs. Since it is becoming increasingly clear that the pattern of opportunistic HIV-associated infections in women is very different from that seen in men, crucial research into women's health issues is being neglected.

It takes little imagination to recognize that, even if HIV infection becomes medically 'manageable', or if a broad enough and safe enough range of therapies becomes available to treat all the opportunistic infections associated with HIV/AIDS in any individual, the problem is far from solved. The necessary drugs will probably be as much out of the reach of disadvantaged individuals or nations as AZT is now, and infected individuals will in all probability have to be on medication for the rest of their lives, with all the attendant health hazards produced by the treatment. Such individuals will require medical supervision, will need to practise safe sex and will need careful and supportive counselling when deciding whether to have children, whether to breastfeed or whether to travel for work or leisure in countries where adequate health support may not be routinely available. Living with HIV will never be easy.

Implications for health policy

In Britain at present we are going through what has been described as a 'crisis in caring'. Health and social services have been rocked by controversial reorganization and by savage financial cuts. The National Health Service is stretched almost to the point of collapse, and in some areas it is now not even possible to guarantee a hospital bed to an emergency admission. Against this background, the prospect of a steadily growing number of patients with HIV-related illnesses is not a cheerful one. Such patients represent an unusual challenge to medical and nursing care. Some may need to spend months in hospital, may be discharged on recovery from an opportunistic infection, only to return weeks or months later ill with another set of symptoms. Some may need periods of intensive care, some may attend on an out-patient basis for tests and checkups for years. One patient may single-handedly test the resources and skills of several different clinical specialisms during the course of a few months, with a range of conditions from fungal infection to tumours, from disorders of the central nervous system to infections of the gut or lungs. Medical and nursing staff may have to cope with the despair of seeing someone go home well only to be admitted again desperately ill, or of watching young women and men sicken and die. The emotional toll is high; burn-out is common among those caring for PWAs.

HIV/AIDS needs to be seen in perspective. It is not, for example, yet among the great killers. Chronic heart disease (CHD) and cancers still kill far more people annually than HIV does. For example, in 1989 in Britain there were 4,496 women known to have cervical cancer, of whom 2,170 died (and for other cancers, such as cancer of the breast, the toll is even greater). In the same year the *cumulative* total of people known to have AIDS reached 848, of whom 301 had died. It is ironic that the safer sex techniques recommended as protection against HIV (using condoms or non-penetrative sex) could probably have prevented the deaths of many more women from cervical cancer than from HIV/AIDS. HIV/AIDS is just one condition among many which needs resources, and in the current political climate something else will have to lose out in order for those needs to be met. Until 1987, funding allocated to AIDS had come out of the budgets of already struggling local health authorities; it had not been 'special' funding. Now, funding decisions are made further up the management hierarchy, at national level. The financial position of the health service is always seen as one of competition for finite resources. It is understood that more money allocated for kidney transplants means less money for special care baby units. Seldom is the equation set in the context of national priorities as a whole, so that the competition is between the defence budget and the NHS, or between tax relief on company cars and prescription charges.

Despite the fact that the number of people needing care for AIDS-related health problems is relatively low in many regions at present, AIDS *is* a special case. Unlike cervical cancer, it is not able to be cured if caught in the early stages. People who have HIV stay HIV+ (and infectious) for life. Unlike CHD it is infectious, threatening people of all ages from birth to old age. And like both cervical cancer and (to a lesser degree) CHD, we know how to prevent it. We are

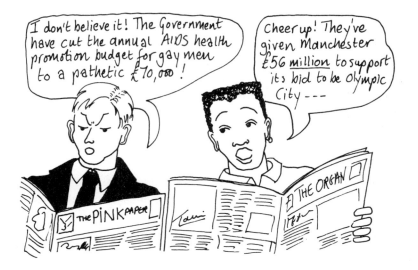

confronted with an epidemic which offers us a very clear choice: to spend now and save later, or to scrimp now and risk our health care system collapsing in the future under the burden of an epidemic such as is now threatening to overwhelm the health care system in New York and other cities in the USA.

Some implications for social services

Because HIV disease strikes people of all ages, social services and care organizations are faced with an unfamiliar and painful scenario. People who need care as a result of HIV/AIDS include those who are sick, which may mean a frail elderly person, an adolescent in local authority care, an orphaned newborn, a young single parent or a middle-aged widower. They also include children left without mother or father, who may be of any age from infancy to late adolescence, and who may be either antibody negative or positive themselves. Such people may come from all walks of life; they may be (one or more of) injecting drug users, professional people or newly released prisoners, those in isolated rural communities or in inner city areas, people from all ethnic, cultural and religious backgrounds, staunch believers in 'traditional' moral codes or politically radical sexual libertarians. Many will bear little resemblance to the stereotypical client of social services.

In order to offer sensitive and appropriate support among such diversity, training and recruitment practices need to reflect an awareness of equal opportunities issues which goes far beyond the superficial. Specialist knowledge of client groups (such as the gay community, refugees or minority ethnic communities) needs to go hand in hand with an awareness of HIV/AIDS issues such as medical care, benefits, housing needs, adoption and fostering, nutrition and the prejudice and discrimination which all too often hound people with HIV/AIDS.

Many of these issues have been recognized and taken on board by social services departments, certainly in those areas where HIV is most commonly found (mainly, though not exclusively, the London boroughs and large urban centres). The British Association of Social

Workers (BASW) has worked to develop strategies for supporting people affected by HIV/AIDS, and to disseminate information widely among its members. Training programmes have been initiated and HIV/AIDS awareness is filtering (with varying degrees of urgency) into the social work courses of colleges and polytechnics.

As ever, the most urgent requirement is for resources. Training programmes require funding and appropriate materials. Establishing specialist HIV/AIDS social work teams (the chosen strategy of many local authorities) requires staff, training, management, and resources such as money to develop specialist reference libraries. National co-ordination requires networking, including mailing newsletters and bulletins and organizing conferences and consultations. All this at a time when social services departments are underfunded, when social workers are leaving the profession and when morale has been shaken by publicly expressed concern about such contentious issues as social workers' handling of child sex abuse. The stressful and often upsetting nature of HIV/AIDS work can only add to the problems of a profession which frequently feels as if it is under siege.

Social services departments have been the instigators of some of the best and most imaginative work for those affected by HIV/AIDS, but they will be called upon in future years to support increasing numbers of people. Even if transmission of HIV were to cease tomorrow, there are still almost certainly thousands of people who have yet to realize they are infected, and there is no suggestion that the epidemic in the UK has 'peaked' yet. With local government finances suffering the slings and arrows of government whimsy over the poll tax and its proposed replacement, funding for social services is under stress at a time when it is essential to establish a firm base for HIV/AIDS work.

Saving lives or saving face? Dilemmas for education

AIDS represents a particularly thorny problem for educational policy. There can be no doubt that the approach taken to date by most schools in the UK can only be described as one of over-caution if not downright cowardice. During 1990 the National AIDS Trust carried out a series of

'Youth Forum' consultations across England to establish what was happening in HIV/AIDS education in schools and also what young people felt they needed. Results were damning. There was an almost universal agreement that education about sex in general, and HIV/AIDS in particular, was inadequate, inappropriate and haphazard. A picture emerged, as NAT moved from place to place, of teachers too embarrassed, too ignorant or too scared of losing their jobs to give their pupils the information they needed to protect themselves from sexual exploitation and abuse, pregnancy, STDs and HIV/AIDS. Given the current chaotic state of central government educational policy with regard to sex education, this is hardly surprising.

There is little public debate, though much private disagreement, about whether or not the state education service should take it upon itself to promote a specific moral code. In a secular and multicultural society such as the UK's, schools serve families which are Protestant, Roman Catholic, Hindu, Sikh, Muslim, Buddhist, Jewish, Methodist, atheist, agnostic, humanist or Rastafarian, along with those from many other minority religious and philosophical groups such as Jehovah's Witnesses or Scientologists. Young people attending UK schools come from a diverse mix of family backgrounds. Some may be living with a lone mother or lone father, some in complex families made up of biological and non-biological parents, siblings and step-siblings. Others may live in households comprising large extended families, with grandparents, uncles and aunts or cousins. Some may come from local authority care, from children's homes or from foster homes. Some may live with adoptive parents, some with their biological mother or father in a lesbian or gay household. A decreasing number will come from the 'traditional' family of biological mother married to biological father, with one or two siblings.

Yet this diversity, far from being reflected in state education policy, is actively *resisted*, especially in the area of sex education, where Britain seems to lag far behind the rest of Europe. There has been a kind of polite war taking place in the arena of school sex education for years, with occasional and bloody skirmishes reaching a wider public through the sensationalist pages of the tabloid press. The two opposing sides are made up on the one hand of those whose job it is to provide and oversee sex education (teachers, Family Planning Authority trainers and experts, Her Majesty's Inspectorate) and those who have a political and ideological agenda (Her Majesty's government, political and religious pressure groups such as the Muslim Educational Trust or Family and Youth Concern). By a depressingly familiar piece of political legerdemain the professionals have been made to appear as the manipulative 'baddies', promoting a left-wing political and ideological agenda in schools, while the real-life politicos and ideologues have acted the part of advocate for the ordinary family, disguising their straightforwardly political motivation beneath a cloak of concern for 'decency'. Thus the government has taken it upon itself to try and oblige schools to inculcate one particular strand of moral and ethical ideology and to denounce all others. This it has done by insisting that Christian assembly and religious instruction remain as statutory obligations in state schools, that sex education be placed in the hands of school governors (a body which it assumes to be composed of its own 'natural' allies), and that where sex education does take place it should be carried out according to government guidelines.

This has resulted in teachers finding themselves in an insecure and often contradictory position from which to educate about HIV/ AIDS. On the one hand, Her Majesty's Inspectorate recommends that:

> the image of society presented in LEA institutions should unobtrusively include same-sex households and affectionate and caring relationships between members of the same sex. Exclusively heterosexist assumptions should be challenged.
> ... approved resources and materials suitable for helping young children understand that human relationships can occupy a range of sex roles should be made available to primary schools.
> ... with regard to all LEA institutions ... disapproval should be expressed at name-calling or physical harassment based on sexual orientation or non-stereotypical sex roles. (from the *Report of the Inspectorate Working Party on Personal Relationships and Health Education, Including Sexual Identity*, 1985)

On the other hand, the Department of Education and Science (DES) insists in a circular sent to all schools in September 1987 that 'There is no place in any school in any circumstances for teaching which advocates homosexual behaviour, which presents it as the "norm" or which encourages homosexual experimentation by pupils'; while the teachers' handbook accompanying the 1988 DES AIDS Education video, *Your Choice for Life*, instructs teachers that:

> It is not sufficient for schools to remain neutral: pupils should understand that the best way for them to avoid AIDS is to refrain from sexual activity until, as adults, they establish a stable, loving and mutually faithful relationship ... The central role of marriage in sexual relationships must be emphasised.

It is hardly surprising that young people are angrily claiming that they have been denied the basic information about HIV/AIDS which they need. It would be a brave and foolhardy teacher indeed who would be prepared to risk providing sensitive and appropriate AIDS education in what amounts to a climate of fear, and the proposed reorganization/privatization of Her Majesty's Inspectorate will do nothing to allay their anxieties. A particularly unpleasant characteristic of establishment 'guidelines' or legislation in this field is the nebulous and ambiguous wording. Faced with the absurd but frequently expressed tenet that simply to recognize the existence of something nasty (sex outside marriage, homosexuality, injecting drug use) is tantamount to unleashing mass, uncontrollable adolescent 'experimentation', and with the equally absurd assertion that young people will never learn to behave in a responsible and moral fashion *unless you explicitly teach them how to do so*, teachers are trapped. Most of them recognize that what they are being told is rubbish; after all, nobody knows better than a teacher just how unpredictable is the link between teaching, learning and behaviour. But there is no dictator more dangerous than an illogical dictator, and 'advocating homosexual behaviour' could mean something as simple as remarking in a music lesson that Benjamin Britten and Tchaikovsky were homosexual, or studying Gertrude Stein's novels or Adrienne Rich's poetry.

The results of all this bizarre confusion are truly alarming. Teenage pregnancy rates are on the increase, a chilling indication that safer sex is not being widely adopted among young people.

Research carried out at Christchurch College in Canterbury shows that school-age young people (especially young men) are extremely anxious and vitriolic not only about gay men and drug injectors but about people with HIV/AIDS: '"They should kill people with AIDS", ... "The people who have AIDS should be shot" ... "The gay bastards spread AIDS and if I catch them I'll cut there [sic] dicks off and kick the shit out of them", ... "My views on AIDS are that there should not be gays", ... "bisexuals ... are the real murdering culprits for introducing the disease into the innocent heterosexual world who are now paying for their filthy behaviour"' (reported at the third Social Aspects of AIDS Conference at South Bank Polytechnic, London, February 1989). Juxtaposing viciousness such as this with the information from the London Lesbian and Gay Teenage Group that a quarter of young gay men are beaten up because they are gay and that one in five young lesbians and gay men are driven to attempt suicide (some succeed), it is clear that the education policy of the Conservative government has not only failed to prepare all young people adequately to protect themselves and others from HIV infection; it has also betrayed thousands of young and vulnerable women and men at the time in their lives when they most need support and validation.

Lessons for schools

So what needs to be done? This is not a question which has ever lacked answers. Groups such as the Family Planning Association, the National AIDS Trust, Her Majesty's Inspectorate and the New Grapevine sex education project in London (now, predictably, defunct after a sudden withdrawal of funds) have all made recommendations about local and national AIDS education policies in schools. The central recommendation of those who are experts in HIV/AIDS education, in sex education, in health education and in teaching young people is that information about HIV/AIDS can only work if it is separated from a moral/political agenda. Young people are not stupid. They know when they are being sold out, they can recognize what is happening when adults take advantage of illness and death in order to try to scare them into 'being good', and they are quite likely to reject the grains of truth along with the moral propaganda. As many educators professionally involved in the practicalities of AIDS health promotion agree, young people must be given sensitive and explicit information, they must be steered away from the anti-gay prejudice which is so damaging to gay and straight alike, and they must be supported in making their own decisions about how best to protect themselves and those close to them from HIV. In particular, the power imbalance between young heterosexual women and men demands urgent attention. It is not enough to repeat meaningless and evasive phrases about assertiveness training for young women while refusing to tackle the real problem – the attitudes and behaviour of young heterosexual men.

As long as the education of our children is bound up with a political agenda, however, such recommendations are just so much wasted breath and printing ink. As a society we are faced with an urgent decision, and one which will not take much more brushing under the carpet. Which is more important: that our children survive and thrive (including those of them who will be lesbian or gay) or that we continue teaching them to hate? For that is what the debate boils down to.

Welfare policy

In some major cities in the USA it is no longer an unusual sight to see a person with AIDS begging in the street. Monetarist economic policy has resulted in a dramatic increase in the extent of poverty in the USA, and AIDS is just another tragedy which follows hard on the heels of deprivation. In Britain we reassure ourselves that the safety net of welfare provision is there to prevent the worst cases of dire and hopeless poverty. But we are kidding ourselves. In London in February 1991 I was confronted by the sight of a young man, with a clumsy cardboard sign hanging on his chest indicating that he was ill with AIDS, half-collapsed against the wall of an Underground subway, begging. He told me that he had been discharged from hospital only to find that his landlord had emptied his belongings out of his flat and moved in another tenant, and that he was homeless, jobless and destitute. The stigma of AIDS magnifies the already serious welfare problems caused by the epidemic.

Lesbians and gay men are no strangers to involuntary homelessness. Many are thrown out of their homes when they make the decision to be honest with their families about their sexuality, or if a landlord discovers they are homosexual. The draconian cuts in benefit rights introduced by the Thatcher administration force young people into prolonged financial dependence on their parents and make it more likely that young women and men who are thrown out of the parental home will resort to begging or prostitution in order to survive. Because there is no legislation protecting the rights of those who are lesbian or gay or who have AIDS, it is perfectly legal to refuse them accommodation, evict them or sack them on the grounds of their sexuality or HIV antibody status. Benefits available to PWAs are pitifully inadequate, making it impossible for them in many cases to afford health-promoting diets, sufficient heating or extra laundry which may be needed. In addition, benefit regulations are designed to deter claimants, being complex and time-consuming, and many PWAs simply do not have the energy and strength required to plough through the bureaucracy. It is not uncommon for the process to take so long that entitlement to specific benefits is not recognized until after the claimant has died.

Homelessness is a national crisis. Homelessness is particularly unforgivable when it hits the vulnerable: those discharged from mental institutions under the 'care in the community' programme, young people rejected by their parents, people who are chronically sick. For people who have HIV or AIDS, homelessness not only is a cause of unimaginable personal misery but represents a very real shortening of survival time. For a society trying to stop an epidemic of HIV/AIDS, homelessness, with the attendant risks of prostitution and drug use, represents a real hazard. It is a short-sighted policy which is based on a belief that society can be strengthened by ignoring or punishing the weak and vulnerable. It is both murderous neglect and dangerous folly to court the wealthy voter with tax cuts while withholding the most basic necessities of life from the young, the unemployable and the sick. Once again, AIDS slides into place within an unjust structure, and once again it is clear that those who condone such injustice are the epidemic's best friends.

A strong and generous welfare benefits system is not a luxury, something to be set up with whatever is left over after the economically productive have been rewarded. It is not just the hallmark but the only guarantee of a strong society. In what are still probably the early days of an epidemic, proper welfare benefits and protected rights to housing, employment and health care for people with HIV/ AIDS represent not just the only possible 'civilized' response but also the best assurance of containing the epidemic. While PWAs have to beg on the streets, we have not yet begun to fight AIDS.

Economic issues

As the recession continues to bite and unemployment to grow, the labour market shrinks at both ends. It is a lucky youngster who leaves school for employment rather than one of the proliferating varieties of 'training scheme'. It is a lucky 50-year-old who can find a new job after redundancy. Early retirement is becoming more common, part-time work is the only expanding sector of the labour market, and fixed-term contracts are commonplace in every type of work, from polytechnic lecturing to pipe-laying. People are also living longer. After retirement, many can expect another twenty years or more of life. The end result of all this is that a decreasing proportion of the economically active are having to support an increasing number of the economically inactive. Add to this the policies of the Conservative administration which have drastically reduced the money available to meet the basic needs of the unemployed, the elderly, the chronically sick or disabled and the very young in order to fund tax cuts for the well off and the outright wealthy, and you have a recipe for disaster. Slot an epidemic of HIV into this scenario and the potential for economic chaos simply becomes that much greater.

HIV is unusual in that, as a sexually transmitted infection, it primarily affects people in young adulthood. People typically become infected in their 20s or 30s, with a growing number becoming infected in adolescence. Given the unusually long asymptomatic incubation period of HIV, people then go on to become sick at any time from a few months to eight or ten years later. In other words, people are becoming ill and dying during a time in their lives when they are at their most economically productive and when they are likely to have dependent children. This means that a possible 'worst case scenario' for a large-scale HIV/AIDS epidemic is catastrophic. In some countries in sub-Saharan Africa, where whole families have been wiped out and entire villages affected, the very old and the very young are left to care for each other.

It takes little imagination to recognize that Britain's recent social and economic policy has left precious little margin for coping with the realities of a steadily growing epidemic. Not only does HIV place a heavy burden on already struggling health and welfare services, but it threatens to exacerbate an already existing structural imbalance in the economy. Not only do those most at risk from HIV represent the most productive sector of the workforce, but they also make up the informal infrastructure of care upon which our society depends. How will we cope when the women caring for their frail elderly relatives, their young children, their disabled family members become ill or die and can no longer care? How will we respond if the breadwinner who has fed and maintained a large family can no longer do so? And what impact will the growth of the epidemic have on our social mores? In the contacts columns of the US gay press, HIV antibody status is often announced; how long will it be before a negative test result is required for a man or (more likely!) a woman to be regarded as marriageable? How long before an HIV test is the nerve-wracking but commonplace precursor to a decision whether to have children or not?

The possible futures for women may be particularly grim; already there are reports of women with HIV infection in Britain and in the United States being pressured into terminating pregnancies or told they must never have children, while others have been refused terminations by ill-informed medical staff unwilling to accept the risk to themselves of carrying out the procedure. For women of colour, aware of the widespread sterilization abuse of Black, Native American and Puerto Rican women in the USA and the on-going dumping of dangerous contraceptives in the third world (see *The*

Black Women's Health Book, edited by Evelyn White), HIV becomes another potential threat to reproductive rights. Yet even privileged, well-to-do white women living in London or Edinburgh are not exempt from the stigma attached to AIDS. This has all been happening in Britain during the 1980s and early 1990s. What will happen in the long term as the epidemic becomes more visible?

There is a feeling of complacency in some quarters, born of the realization that the pessimistic predictions made in the early days of the epidemic have not materialized. The number of recorded cases of AIDS has not matched the very high predictions made five or six years ago, and many people have seized on this as proof that the scope of the epidemic has been exaggerated out of all proportion for political reasons. The epidemic, they claim, does not represent a threat to 'normal' people. This dangerous short-sightedness springs from a quite incredible insularity and stubbornly ignores the evidence of countries such as the United States or Malawi, where the epidemic is more entrenched than it is in Britain (yet). We quite simply have no means of knowing how bad it will get in Britain. In twenty years' time we will probably be laughing at some of the 'worst case scenarios' outlined above. What we do not know, and what we cannot know, is whether we will be laughing because such predictions turned out to be alarmist or because they were too optimistic by half.

How to be an AIDS activist

What is certain is that the sensible thing to do is to plan as far as possible for the worst, not to shake our heads smugly and declare that the whole thing is so much hype. This epidemic, whether it continues to grow or whether we succeed in slowing it down, is *not* under control and is *not* going to go away or burn itself out. It is obvious that the popular press has taken it upon itself to urge its readers to respond to the risk of HIV by casting disdain and contempt upon 'junkies' and 'poofs' and by insulting the Princess of Wales. None of these has any prophylactic value whatsoever. It is equally obvious that central government is prevented from developing an effective response to AIDS by political expediency, particularly when that government is a right-wing one committed to a narrow and moralistic ideology and calling for its support on an unpleasant mix of pseudo-Christian fundamentalism and revivalist imperial nationalism. The loutish and ridiculous determination to make Britain great again is killing Britons just as effectively as the wars of colonialism, only this time they are dying from neglect and bigotry.

AIDS may be a new medical syndrome, but its effects within the body politic are old hat. As we have repeatedly seen, AIDS taps into all the rickety old structures of oppression and injustice. Medically, we have known for a long time how to stop the spread of HIV; AIDS is an epidemic which depends on our denial, our bigotry, our fear, our lack of imagination and our complacency. Amid all the uncertainty about numbers, cures and time-scale one thing is absolutely certain, and that is that none of us can afford not to be an AIDS activist. At the moment, AIDS is in a kind of ghetto, cut off by increasing specialization and professionalization from the mainstream of life. At the moment, people divide up into those who know they are affected by HIV/AIDS and those who still believe themselves unaffected. It is only a matter of time, if we go on behaving as we are doing, before the first group grows to include the latter, as family members, friends and acquaintances become infected or sick. But if we wait for that to happen, we stand very little chance of bringing the epidemic under control. What is needed is an imaginative and informed response *now*.

AIDS activism does not mean you have to chain yourself to the railings outside 10 Downing Street. As Cynthia Chris and Monica Pearl, members of ACT UP New York, write in their conclusion to the book *Women, AIDS and Activism*:

> you don't have to shout at a government building and get arrested to be an activist. Activism on many issues can take many forms. Informally exchanging safer-sex information in a conversation with a friend, or pointing out the bigotry in a colleague's remarks, or questioning what you hear on the news from a government official ... are all forms of activism.

The two keys to AIDS activism are (a) accepting that HIV is *not* something which will go away or which only affects other people and (b) recognizing that fighting AIDS is inseparable from fighting the familiar oppressions on which the epidemic rides. Accepting that HIV exists, that it is a mindless, motiveless virus (not some form of divine or natural retribution for certain minority practices) and that it can hang around for a very long time before making you ill is the first step to fighting it. The next step is getting the information you need about safer sex and/or safer drug use and passing it round to everybody who needs it. You may want to talk to your children about it, your friends and family or your colleagues at work. You may need to work hard to convince yourself, let alone anyone else, that you really do need to take this seriously. You may also find comforting illusions (I'm too old to worry about this ... I'm safely married and trust my spouse absolutely ... I sowed my wild oats before HIV was heard of) extremely painful to confront. But however politically astute or intellectually enlightened we may be, accepting risk and taking responsibility on a personal level is crucial.

The more obvious forms of activism are legion. Writing to MPs to demand better government intervention, organizing within a community to devise appropriate educational materials, making sure you/your children get the information you/they need at school/college, protesting against bigoted and inaccurate reporting in the local and national press, getting condom machines installed in the cloakrooms at work, requesting AIDS training from your union, devising equal opportunities policies which include lesbians, gay men and people with HIV/AIDS, working for your local AIDS organization, donating money to groups which provide services for people with HIV/AIDS, asking your church/synagogue/chapel/temple/mosque to have a collection, hold a special service or pray for people with HIV/AIDS and those working with them, bringing the issue up at your club, coffee mornings, Women's Institute, Young Farmers Club etc. etc., demonstrating against public examples of bigotry (such as Texaco's ruling that all potential employees be tested for HIV) ... the list is endless.

Towards sense in social policy

Personal activism is important, but there is a real risk that by restricting our response to the personal we are feeding into the New Right ideology which sees health and health care as purely a matter of individual responsibility. Successive Conservative governments have ignored or suppressed the steadily growing body of scientific evidence linking poverty and deprivation with ill health and premature death. We are now in the sad position where health is seen as a commodity to be bought and invested in (through private health care schemes) and where hospitals and general practitioners are being forced to compete in the marketplace as though health were no more complex than turnips, and good health care were less fundamental a human right than share ownership.

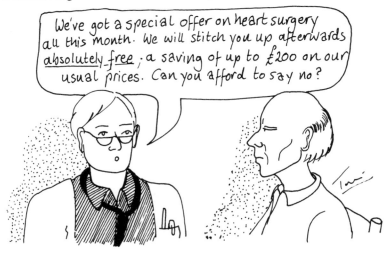

In such a climate, the extraordinary work which is being done for PWAs in the non-statutory sector should be an inspirational example of good practice. If a young white man with AIDS is able to get sensitive counselling at the time of diagnosis, respectful and appropriate medical care at a specialist centre such as the Mildmay Mission or London Lighthouse, support from peer groups, buddies and trained counsellors, advice on safe sex, access to specialist drop-in centres for advice on benefits, legal matters or nutrition and finally terminal care in a specialist hospice, so should a middle-aged Sikh woman with incurable cancer, an elderly West Indian man with Alzheimer's disease, a young Welsh mother with muscular dystrophy. So, indeed, should all people with AIDS; care of this high quality is as yet only available to a minority of PWAs. Such care should not be left up to voluntary organizations funded by insecure local and central government grants and by charitable donations. Good health care is a fundamental right, not a luxury, and is one of the foundation stones of a just society. Faced with all the unknowns of HIV/AIDS, good health care is vital in our struggle to bring a worldwide epidemic under control.

Return to the global village

One of the enduring (if unfashionable) insights of the 1960s was that the destinies of nations may not be separated; the communications revolution and the legacy of colonialism mean that we have to recognize the realities of world economics and world politics. The artificially high standard of living of the affluent (over)developed nations is made possible by maintaining the desperate poverty of the third world (multinational manufacturers supply the well-paid workers of the affluent nations with cheap luxuries such as electronics goods and coffee by paying workers in developing countries poverty-line wages). Trade is already a global structure, with disused Russian battleships being sold by British brokers to ship-breakers in India, who pay their barefoot labourers a few pence a day, ignoring expensive health and safety regulations, to dismantle the huge structures by hand for scrap metal.

Health too is a global matter. Intercontinental flights transport pathogens around the planet swiftly and effectively, with the result that HIV has spread faster and further than any epidemic in history. If we are to be effective in our fight against AIDS, we must recognize and respond to it as a worldwide epidemic. It is simple folly to believe that there is such a thing as 'British AIDS' which is significantly different from 'American AIDS' or 'African AIDS'. If we allow our insularity and prejudice to prevent us taking in the lessons which other countries have so painfully absorbed, we may have to learn the hard way what the World Health Organization and others have been trying to tell us for years: there is *no* group which is not a 'risk group' for HIV infection.

As part of the global community, we in the affluent nations cannot afford to ignore the epidemic in the third world. It is not good enough for a vaccine to be developed in America or Japan if it is too expensive for a state hospital in the Congo or for a family on welfare in New York. That will not stop the epidemic, it will just change its pattern of spread. It is not good enough to allow political parties, religious groups or moral crusaders to 'capture' the epidemic in an attempt to force obedience to their own ideology. That will not stop the epidemic, it will just increase the rate at which it spreads. It is not good enough to allow concerned others to 'take care of' AIDS within discrete medical specialisms or within the non-statutory sector, in the hope that the epidemic will remain neatly confined from the mainstream. That will not stop the epidemic, it will simply weaken our ability to deal with it as 'concerned others' burn out or move on, and the knowledge and experience needed to fight AIDS circulates within a small and marginalized field. It is not good enough to depend on the classic Thatcherite ideology of individualism and every man for himself; there is not much point in sticking to safer sex, saying 'no' to drugs and having your own blood stored in case you ever need a transfusion if the neighbours firebomb your house because there is a rumour going round that your son has AIDS, or you get beaten up in the street because a bunch of homophobes think you look gay, or you get quarantined anyway under some law passed when you were busy being personally responsible and letting other people deal with the politics. A personal responsibility which does not extend to making the world a safer place for people with AIDS, to eradicating prejudice and bigotry or to destigmatizing HIV infection will in the long run backfire.

Conclusion ... for now

HIV is a fragile, highly specialized virus. It is theoretically easy to avoid infection. However, this virus has found human society a particularly accommodating host. It spreads through penetrative sex? We have offered it a culture which iconizes penis–vagina sex and demonizes penis–anus sex, which idealizes the male and degrades the female, thus ensuring that women cannot protect themselves against HIV because they are largely powerless to refuse penetration, and that gay men cannot protect themselves against HIV because they are so stigmatized for their 'contamination' of masculinity that they are denied their basic rights. We have also offered it what every invader needs, secrecy. So anxious about sex are we, so determined to deny it in ourselves and stamp it out in others, that we are simply unable to pass on the accurate and explicit information we all need. It seems we would rather watch our children die than even appear to 'condone' their sexual behaviour.

It spreads through sharing drug-injecting equipment? We have available a population of drug users so marginalized and despised that we are prepared actively to deny them the means to protect themselves from infection, by making it extremely difficult, if not impossible, for them to get clean equipment. It flourishes in those whose resistance is lowered by malnutrition, other infections and diseases? We have enormous numbers of people (even in the wealthiest countries) from whom we have withheld the benefits of modern health care and who struggle from day to day to feed themselves and their families. What is more, we do not take such people very seriously, so we will not do much even when they sicken and die in great numbers.

I said at the beginning of this book that AIDS is a searchlight which throws into sharp relief the good and the bad in our society. There is no doubt that extraordinary and wonderful things are there to be seen. The altruism and responsibility of many (not all) gay men and lesbians, the impressive speed with which medical research dug out the facts about the virus and the syndrome, the speed with which non-statutory AIDS organizations have mushroomed, the willingness of some local authorities (not all) to respond appropriately and effectively, the readiness of certain television networks to take risks and open up debates around sex and sexuality, the courage of many people living with HIV/AIDS who have poured precious energy into the fight against the epidemic; the list is a long one.

However, there is much to be ashamed of, much to be angry about. Medical interest was slow to get started, unwilling to devote energy to something which appeared to affect 'only' gay men and to offer no kudos or financial reward. The medical industry now, policed though it undoubtedly is by AIDS activists, continues to exploit the tragedy of AIDS for profit, while the political and religious establishments of almost every nation in the world continue to exploit AIDS for their own political and ideological ends. The press in Britain, with an international reputation for gay-bashing, continues to feed its readers a deadly diet of homophobia and misinformation, putting the lives of gays and straights alike at risk. The Conservative administration in Britain, committed during the Thatcher years to robbing the poor to pay the rich, devastated health and welfare provision, seemingly content to watch the steady growth in the numbers of people living on or below the poverty line, the numbers of homeless and of those facing the possibility of a lifetime's unemployment. Faced with an epidemic which strikes at the root of their dearest principles, they simply set up endless committees, while offloading the greater part of their responsibility on to the voluntary sector.

Gay men, while taking responsible and compassionate care of their own and working to educate heterosexuals, have shown little willingness to challenge the racism and misogyny which are as much part of AIDS work as homophobia. The traditional forums of radicalism, the women's movement and the left, have on the whole maintained a peculiar silence on the politics of AIDS, punctuated by the odd article in *Spare Rib, New Statesman/Society* and *Rouge*. It is hard to avoid the depressing conclusion that the central question about HIV/AIDS and society may simply be 'So, what's new?'

Appendix 1   Safer sex

HIV is present in infectious quantities in semen. It is also present in fluids secreted by the cervix/vaginal walls. It is important to prevent these fluids getting into the bloodstream, which they can easily do if semen is deposited in the vagina or the anus. There is also a risk from vaginal fluids entering the urethra via the glans of the penis. Safe sex, then, is any activity which does not include penetration by the penis. (This is why lesbian sex is low-risk sex.) So to be safe, stick to variations on mutual masturbation. If this sounds a little limited, perhaps you need to rise to the challenge by introducing variety – rediscover the forgotten joys of dry humping or heavy petting, perhaps? Try playing with baby oil, surgical gloves, chamois leather, silk scarves, feathers or vibrators. The irony of safer sex is that many activities commonly regarded as perverse, such as bondage, are less risky in terms of HIV infection than 'normal' penis-in-vagina intercourse. Now is the time to start talking about how we give each other pleasure, rather than depending on the old familiar routine. Could be the start of something wonderful.

But what about oral sex?

Although the virus has been isolated from saliva, it is not present in sufficient quantity to make saliva an effective source of infection, and no instances of HIV transmission through kissing have been recorded. Semen in the mouth is generally accepted to pose a much lower risk than in the vagina or anus, though there are instances where oral sex does seem to have resulted in transmission of the virus. If a man suspects or knows that he has HIV, it is advisable for his partner to use a condom when sucking his penis. When using a condom for oral sex, wash the lubricant off (it tastes foul) and disguise the taste of the rubber with jam, yoghurt or champagne (you should be so lucky). Do test your preferred substance on a sample condom beforehand ... some surprising foodstuffs weaken or dissolve the latex.

Cunnilingus (licking or sucking the vulva and clitoris) is regarded as a reasonably low-risk activity, though if a woman suspects or knows that she has HIV, her partner should use a latex barrier stretched over the vulva before cunnilingus. Dental dams are recommended for this: originally designed for use by dentists (during dentistry, not sex), they have been widely adopted as a safer sex aid and are now available by mail order. The National AIDS Trust or your local AIDS help line should be able to tell you details of your nearest supplier. It is one of the other ironies of safer sex that dental dams have been promoted exclusively for lesbians, as though heterosexuals never ever had cunnilingus.

Whatever turns you on

It is impossible to say definitively that a particular sexual activity is absolutely safe or that it will definitely result in the transmission of HIV. All that can be said is that some activities are low risk and others high risk. Bearing that in mind, all the following practices carry some degree of risk, though none are as risky as unprotected penile penetration (doesn't that sound romantic): rimming (licking/kissing the anus), fisting (inserting a hand in the rectum or vagina), watersports (playing with urine), scat (playing with faeces), sharing sex toys used for penetration (a dildo or butt plug), sadomasochism (inflicting physical pain for sexual pleasure). Although many of these are relatively safe in terms of HIV transmission, they do carry other health risks. Rimming can result in bacterial or amoebal infections, vaginal fisting has been (unsurprisingly) known to cause injury and infection, while anal fisting can cause peritonitis and even death. Playing with urine is unlikely to cause trouble (some quite well-known people swear that drinking your own urine is a great boost to health and well-being), though it can cause problems if it gets in your eyes, and it should *not* come into contact with the vagina or rectum. The health hazards involved in scat are fairly obvious, including parasitic, bacterial and viral infection. If sex toys are used for penetration, they should not be shared unless they are washed in hot soapy water between users or used with condoms (change the condom between users). Sadomasochism (S/M) is only potentially risky in terms of HIV if blood is spilt; other health hazards may include physical injury or infected scratches.

Real sex?

We are unlucky enough to have grown up in a culture which insists that the only 'real' sex is penile penetration. Everything else (and that often includes female orgasm) comes under the heading of 'foreplay'. It is, therefore, not easy to give up penetration. Additionally, of course, many couples (though by no means all) find it a highly pleasurable and emotionally intense experience, and this is as true of heterosexuals as it is of gay men. There is no way to make penile penetration 'safe' in terms of HIV infection. The best condoms in the world may come off, they may split or tear, a tiny defect may pass unnoticed. Even when used as a contraceptive, condoms are not 100 per cent safe; and there is no 'infertile period' for HIV. Yet it is probably not feasible to expect people en masse to give up penile penetration; the cultural imperative is just too strong.

Using condoms for penile penetration is referred to as 'safer' sex. In other words, it is not safe, but it is much safer than penile penetration without a condom. To be as safe as possible, a few guidelines should be followed. Always buy condoms from a reputable manufacturer, and look for the British Standard Kite mark, or for the Swedish RFSL logo (this is another stringent safety standard). Check the use-by date on the wrapper, as latex disintegrates rapidly over time, and take great care not to damage the condom with finger nails or jewellery when struggling to get it out of the little individual parcels they come sealed in. Pinch the teat between finger and thumb to expel air and leave room for ejaculation (otherwise it may split) and always use a water-based lubricant (such as KY Jelly or Duragel). Some tests have shown that a spermicide called Nonoxynol-9 destroys HIV (which is why it is so widely used as a built-in lubricant on many condoms), but other tests have indicated that it is not particularly good for sensitive human tissue, and there is concern that it may damage vaginal cells. Many women, and some men, are also allergic to it, so it is probably a good idea to use a lubricant which does not have Nonoxynol-9 in it. You can now buy stronger condoms, either for extra safety during vaginal sex or for use during anal sex.

Appendix 2   Safer drug use

Using drugs does not put anyone at risk of picking up HIV. Nor does being addicted to an illegal drug. Nor does injecting a drug (legal or illegal). The only thing which puts drug users at risk for HIV is *sharing injecting equipment*. If you inject drugs, keep to your own equipment. That does not only mean needles, it includes bowls, spoons and syringes – the works, in other words. If you can, get into contact with a needle exchange scheme, where you will be able to get new, unused syringes in exchange for used ones (your local AIDS help line or drugs project will know where your nearest exchange is). Exchange schemes do not put pressure on you to quit, and they will not report you to the police or social services. What they will do is give you clean needles, probably free condoms, and advice about safe sex and HIV testing if you want to know. It is important to remember that many injecting drug users have become infected with HIV through sex, not through their drug use.

If you are in a situation where you have no choice but to share, flush syringes and needles through three times with a solution of ordinary washing-up liquid and then rinse through three times with plain water (otherwise you will end up injecting detergent, which will not do your blood much good). Wash bowls, spoons etc. in the same way. It used to be thought that using bleach was a successful way to clean works, but agencies such as CLASH (Central London Action on Street Health) report that research now suggests that the bleach, rather than killing the virus, simply formed a chemical coating around it. Detergent works by destroying the protein shell around the virus.

The other point to bear in mind is that being high on any drug, whether it is alcohol, ecstasy, cocaine, heroin, marijuana or speed, is likely to affect your ability to practise safer sex. So get into the habit of carrying condoms in your pockets or leave them lying around in the bedroom, to jog your memory.

Further reading and information

If you are especially interested or concerned to find out more about subjects covered in particular chapters, you will find these books helpful. They should all be easily available from good booksellers (even the American ones are titles imported and distributed in this country). If you are told by a bookseller that a particular title is out of print, try your local library. Even if there is no copy in your local branch, they should be able to get you one on loan from another library.

1 No longer someone else's problem

Accessible medical and scientific information about HIV and AIDS can be found in:

AIDS: Scientific and Social Issues by Peter Aggleton, Jan Mojsa, Simon Watney and Stuart Watson (Churchill Livingstone, 1989). This is a slender volume published as part of a training pack, but it is available separately.

The Third Epidemic: Repercussions of the Fear of AIDS (Panos Institute, 1990). Extremely useful facts, figures and information about the virus, transmission, prevention and the global epidemic.

The Terrence Higgins Trust produces a booklet, 'AIDS and HIV – Medical Briefing', which is updated regularly, and which may be obtained direct from: The Terrence Higgins Trust, BM AIDS, London WC1N 3XX.

For information about HIV and injecting drug users, the Institute for the Study of Drug Dependency (ISDD) produces a useful booklet, 'Drugs and Drug Using – A Guide for AIDS Workers', and may also be able to recommend other material. Write to them at: ISDD, 1 Hatton Place, London EC1N 8ND.

2   Fire and brimstone

Material on press and media coverage of AIDS may be found in *Taking Liberties – AIDS and Cultural Politics* edited by Erica Carter and Simon Watney (Serpent's Tail, 1989).

For an assessment of press representation of lesbians and gay men, see *Out of the Gutter – A Survey of the Treatment of Homosexuality by the Press* by Gary Armitage, Julienne Dickey and Sue Sharples (Campaign for Press and Broadcasting Freedom, 1988).

3   Weaker vessels

There is useful information about HIV/AIDS and women in all the following:

Women and the AIDS Crisis by Diane Richardson (Pandora, 1989).

Triple Jeopardy – Women and AIDS (Panos Institute, 1990). This is especially good for the global perspective.

AIDS – Setting a Feminist Agenda edited by Lesley Doyal, Jennie Naidoo and Tamsin Wilton (Falmer Press, 1992). This covers a wide range of issues.

Women, AIDS and Activism by the ACT UP/New York Women and AIDS Book Group (South End Press, 1990). This gives accounts of the situation in the USA, and women's responses.

4   Green monkeys and dark continents

Two books which deal with the issue of racism and AIDS are:

AIDS, Africa and Racism by Richard Chirimuuta and Rosalind Chirimuuta (Pluto, 1987).

Blaming Others by Renee Sabatier (Panos Institute, 1988).

The Panos Institute dossier, *The Third Epidemic* (see above), also contains a lot of useful material on the 'African origins' theory and the effects of racism around the world.

5   Experience and expertise

There has not been a lot written about HIV/AIDS policy in this country. People interested in the statutory and voluntary sector response to the epidemic in the USA are directed to *Reports from the Holocaust* by Larry Kramer (Penguin, 1990).

Anyone interested in policy issues in the UK is advised to investigate the Falmer Press series on the Social Aspects of AIDS, which comprises a series of edited collections of conference papers covering a wide range of HIV/AIDS topics, including policy issues.

There are also articles relating to policy in *Taking Liberties* (see above).

6   Conclusion

AIDS DEMOgraphics by Douglas Crimp and Adam Rolston (Bay Press, 1990). This is an approachable and informative introduction to AIDS activism in the USA.

AIDS – Working with Young People by Peter Aggleton, Chrissie Horsley, Ian Warwick and Tamsin Wilton (AVERT [AIDS Education Research Trust], 1990). This is a training pack for youth and community workers and teachers, but has a full-length introduction to many issues which affect young people and those caring for or working with them. It can be obtained from: AVERT, PO Box 91, Horsham, West Sussex RH13 7YR.

Appendix 1   Safer sex

Making It: A Woman's Guide to Sex in the Age of AIDS by Cindy Patton and Janis Kelly (Firebrand Books, 1987). This gives advice on safer sex and drug use for women, whether heterosexual, bisexual or lesbian.

Safer Sex: The Guide for Women Today by Diane Richardson (Pandora, 1990). This is useful for heterosexual men as well. It attempts to address lesbians and heterosexual women simultaneously, which sometimes does not work, but it is the most thorough guide to safer sex available in mainstream bookshops.

'Haemophilia and Safer Sex – The Choice is Here' (Haemophilia Society). This pamphlet seems to assume there are no gay haemophiliacs, but it is a very useful guide to safer heterosex whether or not you are haemophiliac.

'Lesbians and Safer Sex' by Sue O'Sullivan and Pratibha Parmar (Scarlet Press, 1992).

Appendix 2   Safer drug use

The Terrence Higgins Trust (see p. 155) is the best source of information on drug use and HIV. Other useful information may be had from:

Drugs, Alcohol, Women Nationally (DAWN), Omnibus Workspace, 39 North Road, London N7 9DP (Tel. 071-700 4653).

The Institute for the Study of Drug Dependency (ISDD), 1 Hatton Place, London EC1N 8ND (Tel. 071-430 1991). ISDD has an extensive reference library on drug-related topics, and produces a wide range of useful information, including the magazine *Druglink*, which has regular updates on HIV/AIDS.

Useful addresses and telephone help lines

The Terrence Higgins Trust, 52-54 Gray's Inn Road, London WC1X 8JU (telephone help line 071-242 1010).

The Health Education Authority, Hamilton House, Mabledon Place, London WC1H 9TX (Tel. 071-383 3833).

National AIDS Helpline. This free national help line and information service can offer counselling in languages other than English. The number is 0800 567123, and languages are offered as follows: Cantonese: Tuesday, 6 p.m.-10 p.m., on 0800 282446. Hindi, Gujerati, Punjabi, Bengali, Urdu: Wednesday, 6 p.m.-10 p.m., on 0800 282445. Afro-Caribbean counsellors are available on Fridays, 6 p.m.-10 p.m., on the main number.

Standing Conference on Drug Abuse (SCODA), 1-4 Hatton Place, London EC1N 8ND (Tel. 071-430 2341). SCODA offers advice and information relating to drug use and HIV/AIDS.

London Lesbian and Gay Switchboard. 24-hour help line: 071-837 7324. The Switchboard offers advice and counselling for lesbians and gay men by lesbians and gay men. They can answer general questions about AIDS, and will be able to put you in touch with your local AIDS organizations or your local lesbian and gay switchboard.

The contact numbers and addresses of non-statutory AIDS organizations tend to change. To find out about groups such as Positively

Women, Body Positive, Frontliners, Black HIV/AIDS Network, ACT UP etc., try the Terrence Higgins Trust or the National AIDS Helpline first, as they should be able to give you the most up-to-date information.

Chronology of the UK epidemic

This table provides a very basic outline of the progress of the epidemic in the UK during the first years of the epidemic, and relates this to some important landmarks in the response of the statutory and non-statutory sectors both in the UK and in the USA. Figures are for *reported cases of AIDS*, and are therefore an underestimate of the 'real' number of people with AIDS. Of course, numbers of people infected with HIV will be much higher.

1981

First cases appear in the USA.
Gay Men's Health Crisis born in the USA.
30 cases diagnosed in Europe.

1982

European total reaches 88.
Syndrome now widely referred to as AIDS.

1983

Causative virus for AIDS isolated in Paris ('LAV').
Causative virus for AIDS isolated in USA from French material ('HTLV III').
Agreement reached to name virus 'HIV' (human immunodeficiency virus).
Larry Kramer's article '1,112 and Counting' first published, in *New York Native*.

First safe sex guidelines, 'How to Have Sex in an Epidemic', published by group of gay men in the USA.

Medical Research Council sets up working party on AIDS in the UK.

Friends of Terrence Higgins hold a conference at the Conway Hall, London, out of which the Terrence Higgins Trust (THT) is born.

European total of reported AIDS cases reaches 200.

The USA reports 2,564 *dead* with AIDS.

1984

The THT help line set up, the only source of information available at this time in the UK.

Her Majesty's Customs' 'Operation Tiger' raids community bookshop Gay's The Word in London, seizing 142 titles, including safer sex information and other AIDS-related material. One hundred criminal charges brought against the directors.

European total of reported AIDS cases reaches 685.

1985

The British government makes its first grant to the THT and sets up an Expert Advisory Group on AIDS.

European total of reported AIDS cases reaches 1,729.

1986

The Health Education Council is disbanded and replaced by the Health Education Authority, more directly accountable to central government, and with responsibility for HIV/AIDS education.

The British government targets 'youth' with campaign 'Don't Aid AIDS' in the youth press.

All charges against Gay's The Word directors are withdrawn.

European total of reported AIDS cases reaches 3,518. By now 610 of these are in the UK.

The USA reports 20,000 people with AIDS, of whom 11,000 have died.

1987

President Reagan publicly says the word 'AIDS' for the first time and asks his administration to determine how far the epidemic has spread in the USA.

AIDS Ahead, an AIDS advice and support network for people who are deaf or hard of hearing, is set up with support from the THT. The British government launches 'AIDS – Don't Die of Ignorance' campaign.

Ex gratia payment of £10 million to haemophiliacs infected with HIV via contaminated Factor 8 is announced.

AIDS Coalition To Unleash Power (ACT UP) set up in New York to use direct action to draw attention to political issues around HIV/AIDS and to campaign for improvements in many areas. Other chapters soon mushroom around the USA and begin to grow in European cities.

The British government targets youth press with 'Don't Inject AIDS' campaign.

The overburdened THT accounting system collapses.

The National AIDS Trust is set up in London.

Europe reports 6,533 cases of AIDS, of which 1,227 are in the UK.

1988

Black HIV/AIDS Network (BHAN) set up in the UK.

National media campaign in the UK: 'AIDS – You're as Safe as You Want to Be'.

Section 28 of the Local Government Act, despite mass opposition, becomes law. The Section prohibits the use of local government funds to 'promote' homosexuality, or to represent 'pretended family relationships' as acceptable. A paragraph is tacked on exempting anything carried out to prevent the spread of disease.

European AIDS total reaches 9,199, of which 1,982 are in the UK.

1989

UK Health Departments and the HEA convene a Symposium on HIV and AIDS, to assess progress to date.

UK reported AIDS cases reach 2,830.

Index

with HIV/AIDS, 54-5, 58-9
and misdiagnosis, 58
at risk from heterosexual
    transmission, 58, 59, 61, 65-6
and safer sex, 59-62, 64
and sexuality, 53, 63, 70
as vectors of transmission, 55-7,
    63, 65
as volunteers, 50, 55, 66, 115

Women, Risk and AIDS Project
    (WRAP), 31, 61
World Health Organization
    (WHO), 1, 18, 69, 93, 141
WRAP, *see* Women, Risk and
    AIDS Project
Wrath of God Syndrome (WOGS), 47

Zidovudine, *see* AZT